THE
LAST
TABOO

THE
LAST
TABOO

A SURVIVAL GUIDE TO
MENTAL HEALTH CARE IN CANADA

SCOTT SIMMIE
and JULIA NUNES

M&S

For all the consumers, survivors, and "crazy" people who shared their stories, their strength, and their wisdom.

Canadian Cataloguing in Publication Data

Simmie, Scott
    The last taboo: a survival guide to mental health care in Canada

ISBN 0-7710-8062-X

I. Mental illness – Canada. 2. Mental health services – Canada. I. Nunes, Julia. II. Title.

RA790.7.C3S54 2001   362.2'0971   C00-931819-4

We acknowledge the financial support of the Government of Canada through the Book Publishing Industry Development Program for our publishing activities. We further acknowledge the support of the Canada Council for the Arts and the Ontario Arts Council for our publishing program.

Design by Ingrid Paulson
Typeset in Sabon by M&S, Toronto
Printed and bound in Canada

McClelland & Stewart Ltd.
The Canadian Publishers
481 University Avenue
Toronto, Ontario
M5G 2E9
www.mcclelland.com

1 2 3 4 5   05 04 03 02 01

CONTENTS

FOREWORD

This is an optimistic book about a difficult subject. It confronts the mystery and fear surrounding mental illness, the challenges of accessing appropriate services, and the roadblocks put up by society's attitudes. And it counters these realities with practical solutions, described by the real people who have tried them.

As a guide for leading the reader through the mental health field, *The Last Taboo* is a unique resource which fills a current void. For people unfamiliar with the field, it provides a map of the territory. For individuals who have experienced the mental health world as a consumer, family member, or service provider, it offers not only validation, but new ways of exploring the terrain. It addresses most common mental disorders, although it does not cover some particular conditions such as Alzheimer's disease and related dementia-type disorders.

At the Canadian Mental Health Association, we have learned that there are many different perspectives on the difficulties and solutions, but no single answer. We see the problems every day. They include the complexity of mental illness itself, the stigma and ignorance surrounding it, inadequate services, and insufficient attention to people's quality of life. The obstacles are fairly visible to most of us working in mental health, but sometimes the solutions are harder to come by. Where do we begin?

In fact, the strategies currently in place are almost as complex as the problems. As this book describes, there is the most obvious "formal" system of service providers, medications, and therapy. This is a very important resource to many people, but it is certainly not the only option. There is also an "informal" system of family, friends, and neighbours, and of others who have been through the same experience. It is a very different, but equally powerful, resource. And then there are the regular experiences of community to which every citizen is entitled: "a home, a job, a friend." These, too, are critical elements of hope and recovery.

The people you will meet in the pages that follow put a human face on the many and different routes to healing. Whether it is a person in crisis gaining access to a rigid, unyielding system, a family member finally coming to terms with a long-past suicide, or an executive using alternative therapies, the stories in this book illustrate the many obstacles and paths around them in this field.

Underlying all of these approaches, there is one positive theme that seems to keep emerging. This is the need for control over one's life.

In the past several years, we've become increasingly aware of the importance of control in the various mental health issues we deal with. Employees who have control over the conditions of their work have a better chance of maintaining their physical and mental health than those with little control. People talking about their experiences of recovery from mental illness tend to mention control as a contributing factor. People in all kinds of situations feel better about the decisions which affect them and about themselves if they have control over those decisions.

Scott and Julia's harrowing story about losing control and hope, and the long struggle to get them back, sets the theme for this book. We are shown the many different ways that people have gained control, and tips for navigating the various routes to health. By demystifying mental disorders and providing strategies for dealing with them, this book hands control back to the consumers and families, where it belongs.

In the end, *The Last Taboo* is a practical road map for people with mental disorders and those who care about them. All of us looking for paths to hope and recovery can find encouragement in these pages.

Ed Pennington, General Director
Bonnie Pape, Director of Programs and Research
The Canadian Mental Health Association

ACKNOWLEDGEMENTS

Every story has a beginning. And this book is a direct result of the faith and generosity the Atkinson Charitable Foundation showed back in 1997. That was when the Foundation and its executive director, Charles Pascal, took a chance on a proposal written by a man who'd once been psychotic. Through the Atkinson Fellowship in Public Policy, the Foundation funded a year of research and writing that culminated in the *Toronto Star*'s "Out of Mind" series in 1998.

David Reville was Scott's mentor on that project. He has remained both a friend and supporter, one who wisely told us to smarten up when we (briefly) considered abandoning this work. We're fortunate to have met him. We're also grateful to the *Toronto Star* for its tremendous support, both of the series and this book. Few employers would give someone a leave of absence during their first year on the job to disappear and write. (Unless, of course, they *wanted* them to disappear!)

We thank Doug Gibson at McClelland & Stewart for his encouragement and especially for his patience, which went above and beyond the call of duty. He also gave us some free books, which made us very happy. Our editor, Alex Schultz, offered solid critiques, burned up several erasers, and taught us, a lot, about commas. We taught Alex much about procrastination. Together, we believe we improved this book.

There are many, many people and institutions who gave freely of their time, knowledge, and encouragement. Space, unfortunately, doesn't permit us to name everyone, and we apologize in advance to those we can't mention here.

The Canadian Mental Health Association has been incredibly supportive. Its provincial divisions took the time to fill out a questionnaire regarding mental health resources in their region, which helped form the Appendix. Every single provincial health department in the country did the same thing – and everyone mailed them back! The Mood Disorders Association of Ontario provided access to its library, support group meetings, photocopier, and coffee. Even before this became a book, the Mood Disorders Association of Canada told us to write one.

But you can't write without doing research. The people with the Arthur Sommer Rotenberg Chair in Suicide Studies were tremendously helpful, providing interviews, data, and contacts for the chapter on suicide. The Centre for Addiction and Mental Health hooked us up with some of the most prominent authorities in the field and granted access to their library. Many psychiatrists from outside CAMH were especially generous with their time during our early research. They include doctors Jim Deutsch, Stephen Connell, Sam Malcomson, and Ty Turner.

Others connected with the mental health field were also crucial. People like Ken Ross of New Brunswick, a man instrumental in one of the more progressive mental health systems in the country. The CMHA's Eric Macnaughton was of tremendous assistance in B.C., providing us with some great studies and profiles. Art Gondzolia of the Schizophrenia Society of Saskatchewan helped find us some good prairie people to write profiles. Speaking of which, Barb Wilson deserves a medal. Several of the profiles came, with her assistance, from the outstanding consumer/survivor periodical she edits called *Open Minds*. And, of course, thanks go to *all* the people who graciously agreed to share their stories in this book.

Antipsychiatrist activist Don Weitz, who will probably hate this book, also deserves thanks. Though we don't always agree with Don, we appreciate the volumes of material he supplied. Survivor organizations like the Ontario Council of Alternative Businesses (thanks, Diana) and the Parkdale Recreation-Activity Centre (thanks, Bob) were great, and taught us much about human potential – and the importance of a home, a job, a friend. The Keele Street Women's Group kindly allowed Julia to sit in on meetings rarely open to journalists. And research assistant Brenda Nunes (yup, Julia's mom) was indispensable. She patiently mailed surveys, conducted interviews, typed transcripts, and – on holidays – cooked great meals.

To ensure our chapters hit the mark, we roped in several very busy people to read them. Many of them helped in other ways, too. They include doctors Roger Bland, Jacques Bradwejn, Paula Goering, Paul Links, Jane Murphy, Karen Schonbach, Howard Tanen, Bryan Tanney, and Don Wasylenki. Non-physicians who helped out include Kalyna Butler, Kate Kitchen, and Neasa Martin. Lawyers who read excerpts (but didn't bill) deserve applause: Michael Bay, Suzan Fraser, and Anita Szigeti. And a standing ovation to those who read the entire manuscript and offered comments: the CMHA's Ed Pennington and Bonnie Pape, as well as David Reville and Phil Upshall.

It's sometimes said that only 10 per cent, or less, of your research actually makes it into the final product. We figure we're at about 2 per cent. That means, unfortunately, that scores of people who were interviewed did not make it into these pages. Their input, however, helped shape our views and this book immensely. (Maybe we can get you into the next one.)

Our greatest debt, however, is to those closest to home. Our lives would not be the same without our families, friends, and others who cared. They stuck with us, unflaggingly, through the darkest period of our lives. A special and lasting "thank you" to Lyle, Kathy, Lois, Brenda, and Alex, along with Tom, Daryl, Dianne, David, Steve, and Karen.

CHAPTER ONE

Scott's Story

It can happen to anyone.

And it happened to me.

This is the story of a slow, seductive descent into madness. A fantastic and terrifying voyage through several countries and a number of states of mind. Geographically, it roams from Chechnya to China to Canada. Psychologically, it ranges from indescribable elation to near-suicidal grief. Yet it is, ultimately, a story with a happy ending. Happy, because I survived it.

This is an account of what it is like to be traumatized, hospitalized, stigmatized, and – ultimately – to recover. Of the strain on – and the importance of – family, spouses, and friends during a time of crisis. Of the two-edged sword of powerful psychiatric drugs. Of losing hope forever, only to find that it still existed. Of going to hell. And back.

First off, I'll tell you that my entire career has been in journalism, much of it in Toronto as a senior writer for CBC's *The National*. I also enjoyed brief notoriety as "the voice" that boomed the nightly headlines: "Tonight . . . on *The National* . . ." That was me. (Great gig, that.)

I'd always longed, though, for a foreign posting. And in June of 1994, I got my wish. Moscow Bureau Producer. Basically, that meant working with the correspondent to gather, assemble, and transmit daily news stories. A fairly high-pressure job, but I'd worked in many stressful situations over the years and handled them well. After all, news *is* stress.

My partner, Julia, who is also a journalist, joined me, planning to freelance. Both of us were eager to actually see history being made, rather than watch it flicker by on a television screen. We weren't disappointed: whether it was the crumbling ruble or a stumbling Yeltsin, it was a city, a country, always on the precipice.

Some of the stories our bureau worked on will remain with me always. During a trip to Chechnya months before its 1994–95 war with Russia, a warm and tenacious people opened their doors and hearts to us. Our crew was accorded the privilege of videotaping a Chechen wedding, which was marked by joyful – and repeated – machine gun volleys. Some people throw rice; Chechens like to fire bullets. During the reception, the groom's brother, in a fit of spontaneous revelry, squeezed eight rapid shots from his pistol into the dining room ceiling. Wedding guests, who were dancing in the same room, didn't even blink.

So there was fun stuff. But there was not-so-fun stuff, too.

In late September we travelled to Finland when the passenger ship *Estonia* went down, a tragedy that claimed the lives of 852 people. I flew, with our cameraman, in a Finnish rescue helicopter to the site where the ship lay seventy metres below the surface. As we hovered over the Baltic, an indifferent sea offered no hint of the steel tomb on its floor. Yet I couldn't help but picture the dead forever trapped in that darkened hulk, visualize the panic as the *Estonia* slipped into icy black.

Most journalists are pretty adept at distancing themselves from the pain they witness; it's almost a prerequisite if you're going to survive in the field. I'm pretty good at it, too. But the *Estonia* clung to me like a fog. And then, a couple of weeks later, back in Moscow, the clouds moved in. Literally. Great slabs of slate converged, as if summoned by magic, to blacken the city's skyline.

"Take a good look at the sun," advised Tanya, our office translator. "Because you will not see it again until May."

Russians tend to predict gloom with uncanny accuracy.

By October, the sky was oppressively leaden every day, a reflection of the misery so prevalent in the Russian capital; misery which resonated with nearly every story we covered. Impoverished pensioners. Disorganized crime. Corruption. Conflict.

I had no history, other than one brief depression while on assignment in Thailand, of mental health problems. But as fall became winter, replete with snow that turned black as it fell, I could feel *something* coming on. It became slightly more difficult to get out of bed. My energy level started to drop. I started to want *out* of Moscow, or at least out of that particular position, and began to make it known. The correspondent and I also started getting on each other's nerves – something I had almost never experienced professionally before. But my problems weren't just at the office.

Relationships and commitment had always been issues for me, and I was being true to form. Life in Moscow was complicated immeasurably for Julia and me by the difficulty I was having in adjusting to a monogamous, stable relationship. Part of me wanted out, was convinced I could find greater happiness elsewhere. So there was more on my plate than merely the weather.

Figuring out where all this began becomes something of a chicken-and-egg proposition. Did I start to dip solely because there was much on my mind, or because I'm the type of person who is more susceptible to mood changes? After all, many people endure far worse situations without taking a depressive nose-dive, while others muddle through seemingly lesser trials yet still become mired in despair.

I believe it was a mix of the two – a combination of real-life turmoil with what is often termed "vulnerability." Whatever the mysterious ratio between those two factors, my shift in mood did not come out of thin air. Indeed, when there are *no* serious troubles in my head (which, trust me, is most of the time), I do not become depressed.

Though I knew I was unhappy and dissatisfied, I was not aware that I was truly depressed. Nor did I have time to give the possibility much thought. During December, as renewed tension built between Russia and Chechnya, we filed stories every single day save Christmas (when we were in the bureau anyway). When that tension turned to war, it became clear we would have to go there. Our CBC crew prepared to leave in early January 1995.

I can't speak for other members of the crew, but I was scared. I'd covered just one other major armed conflict during my career, the ill-fated Chinese student movement and resulting Tiananmen Square crackdown. I'd learned then that death looks vastly different in person than it does on television. I'd also had a very close call in Beijing – and the reports we'd been hearing from Chechnya were chilling.

The Russians, it seemed, were not just hunting military targets. In a strategy aimed at terrorizing the populace, the army was also setting its sights on civilians. Public places like markets had already been hit. A young American woman, a Moscow-based photographer, had been decapitated in Grozny during a rocket attack on a central square. Such occurrences give one pause to reflect.

But news is about conflict. And major conflict is major news.

We set up operations in neighbouring Dagestan, where most foreign news operations had based themselves. That meant we'd drive into Chechnya every day, gather our material, then drive back as night fell. Though we did have good flak jackets and helmets, we did not have a good vehicle. The CBC's armoured car was in Sarajevo and could not be transported at such short notice. We were reduced to hiring a local driver and his aging Lada.

It was with a certain feeling of vulnerability, then, that we drove through hostile territory in a car with the structural integrity of a beer can. A vulnerability magnified when Russian jets swooped low, firing rockets. Our only protection was electrician's tape, which we'd used to mark "TB" (Cyrillic for "TV") on the side of our car. It was debatable whether such markings were helpful, or the equivalent of writing "Aim Here!" (An NBC producer told us their vehicle, with similar markings, had been deliberately targeted by a Russian tank.)

Suffice to say it was grim and dangerous work. Adrenalin was on overdrive. Russian air raids in close proximity became, if possible, routine. The threat of cluster bombs – devices containing smaller bomblets designed to fragment and tear through steel and flesh – was omnipresent. We became adept at diving into mud-filled ditches at the first sound of an approaching jet. (Though, due to supersonic speed, those jets had actually passed over by the time you heard them. Meaning that if they *had* dropped bombs in your vicinity, the odds of finding cover prior to impact were pretty slim.) On three separate occasions, I believed my life was in danger.

We witnessed much during our week in the war zone. A market where some fifty people had been killed was still littered with the perforated hulks of their cars, all of which, shredded by shrapnel, looked like bloodied cheese graters. Grozny, the capital city, was being methodically reduced, rocket by rocket, to a gravel pit. Children roamed the craters of former homes, searching for vestiges of their former lives. Trapped civilians roamed the alleys, looking for food and water. Stray dogs roamed the streets, scavenging for corpses.

All this, plus meeting daily news demands. Up early to drive to Grozny; up late with scripts and satellite feeds.

In the days following our return to Moscow, I remained very much on edge. Sharp sounds would cause me to jerk in a startled fashion. Sleep was not as restful. And hearing anything that sounded remotely like a jet – even the whine of a truck transmission – could send a chill up my spine.

I clearly needed a break – and needed to sort out my future with Julia.

I left Moscow for a trip back to Canada feeling so stressed and confused that while in Toronto I sought the counselling of a psychologist through the CBC's Employee Assistance Plan. He said there were two options, depending on how deep these issues ran: longer-term therapy or a concerted effort to move on. I convinced myself the issues could be overcome with sheer willpower, that it would be possible simply to fix my life.

In February I returned to Moscow, to Julia, with determination. Despite the chronically bleak Russian winter, I would make both my posting and my relationship *work*. I resolved to be happier than before, more content than before.

And that was when things started to happen. I began, quite simply, to feel better than normal. Significantly better. The troubled thoughts that had been cluttering my head miraculously began to vanish.

Though unaware of it, I was in the early stages of something psychiatrists call hypomania, a phase of what is known as bipolar affective disorder (or manic depression). Since I'd never experienced this before, I knew only that I felt good. But I was starting to exhibit classic symptoms: decreased need for sleep, grandiose ideas, excessive talking. Though it can sometimes run in families, there was no history of the disorder in my clan. It affects between one and two per cent of the population, and stress is known to be one of many triggers.

There was no doubt I'd been through the most stressful period of my life (so far). But at this stage there was nothing really to indicate – least of all to me – that anything was wrong. I was able to apply myself fully to the job – so fully, that I eagerly tackled a punishing work schedule. In fact, I made it *more* punishing by adding unnecessary tasks.

I also started to think about business ideas. This had long been a pet hobby of mine, but it now became a sideline obsession. I had *good* ideas, and I spent any spare time extolling to colleagues the benefits of wondrous ventures on which we could collaborate.

In this early phase of the disorder, I was enthusiastic. By most accounts fun to be with (though Julia, as you'll see, does not share this assessment). Several colleagues remarked on how happy I now seemed. It only added fuel to the fire.

This energy – and it's really the only way to describe it – did not leave me at night. So, in a form of self-medication common with the disorder, I would pour a Scotch to relax. Then another. It seemed to be the only way I could calm myself to the point where I could sleep. Julia noticed the increase in drinking and expressed concern, but I was quick with an excuse: "Work's been stressful," or "I'm just a little tense." And, of course, it's socially acceptable to drink in Russia; it's an integral thread in the tattered social fabric.

So, there I was. Late at night in our Moscow apartment. Feeling energized, feeling slightly powerful, and – in retrospect – frequently feeling drunk.

And always nearby was my trusty laptop. Equipped with a modem.

That laptop was my link with the CBC computer system, my umbilical cord with Canadian and world news.

It was also dangerous.

A perception that I'd been mistreated by a manager took on new and larger significance. I was starting to develop a somewhat grandiose belief in what I considered long-neglected abilities. Whatever rational editing process normally exists in the brain started going haywire. I'd bash out long notes – with an uncharacteristically defiant tone. And then, without so much as a second thought, press "send."

If I had to pinpoint a time when this disorder was becoming serious, it would be when I first pushed that "send" button.

Of course, management did not take well to receiving impertinent notes from an employee who was suddenly acting like a jerk – an employee who would quickly apologize for those notes, only to fire a new salvo in another few nights. Over a period of several weeks, I succeeded in raising the concern (and likely the blood pressure) of my pen-pal manager. He rather kindly suggested I leave Moscow and return to a different position in Toronto. It seemed, to me, out of the question. Why leave when I was feeling so great – greater than I'd felt in years? I told him that, while I appreciated his concern, I wanted to stay.

The run-in with management ended with an agreement to retain me in my post, subject to quarterly reviews of my performance. I was, in effect, on probation. And that, of course, added additional stress; stress the disorder itself had caused.

Over the next several weeks, the hypomania kept on rolling. I required less and less sleep, would type up long lists of business ideas on the computer, began believing I could achieve anything I set my mind to. And at that stage, I probably could have.

For example, I bought a beautiful antique wall clock that didn't work. Though mechanically inclined, I'm no watch repairman. Nonetheless, I managed to take that entire clock apart in a few hours, determine what was causing the problem, then reassemble it. And it worked. I was some kind of genius. (Actually, it stopped after a couple of days. But it kept perfect time until then.)

During this period Julia and I took a trip to Estonia, where a good friend of mine, a Canadian of Estonian descent, had established a successful business. He liked some of my business ideas. And I certainly liked his. So much so, that I invested many thousands of dollars in his company without a second thought. (It turns out this actually *was* a good investment decision.)

But imagine. Acting on such impulses.

Of course, it's not a rational way to think. Most of us weigh actions against possible consequences before taking the plunge. To me, however, it was an exciting way to think. An exciting way to *live*. So enthralling was this new way of life that I coined a motto to encapsulate its limitless possibilities. I posted a copy of it above my desk and another one at home. It stated: "I know where I am and I know where I'm going." I repeated this phrase often, affirming my belief that I could accomplish anything in life.

The crunch came in early May, during a summit between Bill Clinton and Boris Yeltsin, a meeting that was to cap the fiftieth anniversary of the 1945 Victory in Europe celebrations. These ceremonies, extensively covered by Western media, had started in London and been moving eastward across Europe.

Since Prime Minister Chrétien was to be in Moscow for the celebrations, since our bureau would be filing several stories daily in both French and English, there was a tremendous amount of work to do. Satellite feeds to book. Stories to plan and pre-shoot. Briefing notes to prepare. Logistics to arrange for other CBC staff travelling with the prime minister.

The night those crews arrived, I met them at a late-night hotel briefing. Their equipment, hundreds of kilograms of it, had been delayed at the airport. I volunteered to return to the bureau and await its arrival. It got there around two o'clock in the morning. I helped the bureau driver, Sasha, unload everything, then kept on working. A massive military parade was just hours away. Because I was on probation, nothing could be left to chance. So I worked – excuse the pun – like mad. Sleep was, in my mind, an unnecessary luxury.

After staying up all night, I should have been exhausted. But I was pumped. And despite some tense moments, our coverage that day was solid. My editorial judgment – my news skills – remained intact. In retrospect, the scripts I wrote still look pretty damn good. Some of the best speed-writing I've ever done. (One of them garnered glowing notes of praise from CBC folk back home – positive reinforcement of my boundless talents.)

Which, of course, is a curious thing about this particular disorder.

People – at least in the early stages of hypomania – don't necessarily appear unwell. They are still able to work, in some cases better than before. A colleague from Ottawa would later remark to a friend that he was "in awe" of my organizational skills. But he could also see that I was off-balance in other ways. He thought I was talking non-stop, in his words "acting paranoid."

At home, any questioning of my behaviour was met with vigorous denial. How could anything be wrong when I was doing great work, filing several scripts a day in addition to my planning duties? When, in fact, I was feeling on top of the world?

It would soon start to unravel.

On the last night of the summit, after writing the final script, I snapped. While visiting the nearby Worldwide Television News bureau, I delivered a bottle of vodka to thank the staff for technical assistance. I had a drink while there and, while yakking, made some disparaging remarks about our correspondent. People there made similar comments about our Russian videotape editor. Their words seemed to confirm my belief that our bureau was incompetent.

When I returned to our office, I blew up at the editor in question. I also blew up at the correspondent who'd hired her, demanding to know if the reporter had made a background check prior to making the decision. There was no violence or threat of violence – but I did yell, explosively, making no effort to contain my anger. And that's not like me.

The correspondent phoned senior managers back in Canada and said she'd no longer work with me, that I was behaving "like a madman." They phoned me from Toronto the next day and said I was barred from the CBC's Moscow office pending an investigation. I was also prohibited from having any contact with my fellow employees. I felt betrayed. And isolated. I had no idea I'd done anything wrong.

In my defence, I set out to document all that had happened. Aided by my growing energy, I typed roughly two hundred pages in a two-day period (some people are very productive during this stage). Enough material for a book. My tone was uncharacteristically defiant. I was invincible. I would take on the CBC and win. How could I not? There was, after all, nothing wrong with me.

A producer from CBC London was named the investigator in my case. We met in a hotel lobby to discuss the complaints against me. Though we've never spoken since, the producer must have seen I was paranoid. I told her I was concerned that a bomb may have been planted under the bureau's car (which

I'd driven to the meeting) and asked her to have our drivers check it out. I left the hotel saying I'd feel safer taking the Metro home. And then things *really* got weird.

Outside, I began to wander, guided by some invisible but meaningful hand. I drifted aimlessly through a modern department store until a haunting piece of music by Philip Glass caught my ear. It was synchronized to a massive tower of television monitors, where scenes of nature – mountains, fields, waterfalls – filled the screens. I felt I had come to the right place.

That same gentle presence guided me up a series of escalators. As I rose to the top floor, accompanied by the rhythmic, hypnotic music, I met with the sudden and wonderful realization that Christ would be waiting on the top floor. An internal radiance filled me, one so powerful I thought I would soar. I was also aware of a pleasurable tingling sensation inside the very crown of my head. It felt, for all the world, like something inside my brain was changing. It likely was. I was almost levitating when I reached the top floor.

Christ was not in the furniture department. Oh well. Maybe next time. And just like that I shrugged off this powerful delusion – which moments earlier had been the pinnacle of my existence – as if it were nothing out of the ordinary. Presumably Christ had another appointment in his Daytimer and would catch up with me later. I floated back down the escalator, drinking in the beauty of the music and the accompanying images. The accusations against me were the furthest thing from my mind. It was, even now in memory, a beautiful moment.

I drifted home in this same surreal state. Something would tell me when to get off the subway, when to get back on. I rode several trains, rolling beneath the capital in a highly circuitous route. Hours later, I finally disembarked at a station near our apartment. I felt there was a reason – other than going home – that compelled me to leave the subway at that particular stop. That there was something waiting for me.

I was about to be introduced to a phenomenon psychiatrists call "ideas of reference," the belief that some completely random occurrence is an omen or message intended specifically for you. Their impact on a receptive mind cannot be overstated. For some people, this can be as bizarre as believing a licence plate contains a coded message from aliens. In my case, the special object was a Russian military night-vision scope.

I'd actually looked for one of these, casually, since arriving in Moscow. And barely twenty-four hours earlier, a colleague back in Canada had sent me a note asking if I could find one for him. Imagine my astonishment, then, just a few hours after Christ cancelled, when I discovered someone selling night-vision scopes at the top of the Metro stairs.

What would have earlier been a happy coincidence took on *profound* significance. Significance of what, precisely, I couldn't tell you now. But it felt so overpowering at the time that I was trembling when I made the purchase.

Over the space of the few blocks home, however, that excitement became transfused with trepidation and paranoia. The mafia was out to get me, displeased with some of the stories the bureau had produced. (Moscow is an easy place to be paranoid, because – in a city where mafia murders and bombings are daily fare – people quite often *are* out to get you.) Maybe they would try to get me at night, in the dark. Perhaps I had found this night-vision scope for a reason. Maybe it was intended to save my life.

Julia could not quite follow my twisted logic and looked deeply concerned. The following morning I set out to calm Julia. "Yes, I had overreacted. Yes, there was nothing to it. Yes, it was not like me. Must just be stress." (I didn't really believe I'd overreacted. That scope was special – but I kept that secret to myself.)

Then came judgment day. The results of the investigation were not shared with me. Two managers, on the phone from Toronto, announced only its conclusion: "Your position," I was told, "has been terminated." There was no mention of my mental health, no mention of my job performance, not even any mention of "the incident." In fact, no reason at all was offered for the decision. I was told to return to Canada, take a break, then return to my old job on the writing desk. This was not good news. (In fact, it was astonishing news. I had assumed, after they'd read my brilliant defence, that all would be forgiven. My first words in the conversation were, "How about an apology?" – a query met only by static on the phone line.)

I was also sternly informed that any attempt to publish or disseminate my defence, which critiqued many aspects of the CBC's Moscow bureau, would result in harsh consequences. Were I to ignore that warning, stated one of the two managers, "The entire weight of this corporation will be brought to bear on your shoulders." To say that this freaked me out would be a monumental understatement.

I discovered, during my next attempt to log in to the network, that my messaging privileges on the CBC computer system had been revoked. Though I understand now why this step was taken, I most certainly did not understand then. I was in shock. This was a crisis.

And crises are not good for hypomania. I was, apart from that one sleepless night at the bureau, averaging about four hours a night. After being removed from the post, I slept less. I was now on a collision course with full-blown mania.

Under normal circumstances, what had transpired might give one pause to reflect. I'd been removed from a post I'd worked my entire career to obtain. I'd been ordered to return to a desk job I had years ago grown weary of. Instead, it seemed to rev me up. After about two minutes of shock, I understood this was *meant* to happen. I was destined for greater things. This was my chance to realize my full potential. This was *freedom*.

As part of my now smouldering contract, Julia and I were still owed one trip outside of Russia. So I requested to fly to China, a country for which I feel an incredibly strong bond. Soon we were on a flight to Germany for a connection to Hong Kong and then Beijing.

Changing time zones isn't great for this disorder at the best of times. Disrupting regular sleep patterns can, in some people, trigger an episode and will almost always exacerbate one in progress. In other words, flying an extraordinary distance while hypomanic was probably the worst thing we could have done. (I did, however, have a very happy flight.)

Returning to Beijing was, for me, a profoundly emotional experience. I'd lived in the country more than two years, been in Tiananmen Square the night the army attacked in June 1989. Our trip coincided with the sixth anniversary of that fateful night.

I have many good friends in Beijing, so returning to the capital was a bit like a homecoming. Old colleagues remarked on how full of energy, or Qi, I was. (They would tell me, months later, they had actually been concerned for my health but felt uncomfortable about broaching the topic. Friends back in Canada would say the same thing.)

I likely would not have listened, anyway. I was too consumed with planning my business empire. What I lacked in details I more than made up for in enthusiasm. I recall planning everything from a bagel-and-coffee chain to a Chinese MTV channel. I still have a list of those ideas. Some are good (a Canadian bagel chain has since opened and is thriving in Beijing), the majority hysterical.

This is not atypical of hypomania and mania. Many people in their seductive grip get an idea and just *go* with it, often spending their way to financial ruin. The ability to foresee consequences goes straight out the window, sprouts wings, and flies to Mars. One Vancouver man purchased a personal submarine while manic; I chose antique Chinese furniture.

The aesthetics of century-old Asian furniture have always appealed to me; in fact, I had considered exporting it to Canada back in the late 1980s (when I was fine). But the aesthetic appeal of this stuff when hypomanic was indescribable. The intricacy of carvings. The beauty of a simple chair. The fragrance of camphor wood. Perfection.

Clearly, an export business could not fail. All we had to do was buy the stuff, and the rest would take care of itself. People would be lined up for blocks, buying our furniture and toasting my inscrutable Eastern wisdom with fine jasmine tea. Nothing could be simpler.

When Julia questioned my lack of a concrete business plan, our lack of a store for that matter, I was quick with an enthusiastic response. "We'll sell it from the dock!" I proclaimed, picturing a crowd of eager customers who shared my excitement.

And thus began the shopping. I swept through the antique market like a whirlwind. Something would catch my eye, I'd barter at the speed of light, and the deal would be done. A salesman's fantasy. I spent $5,000 the very first day.

And the next. And the next. Until – $25,000 later – we had an entire forty-foot container load. The precise number of pieces escapes me, but it was more than one hundred – and a huge canopy bed would count as just one.

That's a lot of furniture.

At one point I contacted my Toronto real-estate agent, told him I wanted to purchase a building for the store. The agent, who's a tall, bald guy, is at the top of a very competitive heap. It suddenly dawned on me that he was bald . . . because he was a *Buddhist*! Clearly, this explained his domination of the Toronto condo market. Good idea. Perhaps I, too, should adopt this faith.

I also adopted – temporarily – a new name. When you tell someone in China that you're from Canada, they invariably invoke the name of Dr. Norman Bethune. His Chinese moniker is a clever transliteration of "Bethune": *Bai Chou An*, literally "White Seeking Peace." I told people that, while I was not Bethune, I was indeed a White Seeking Peace. My Chinese acquaintances appeared to think this was quite clever. Believe me, I did.

During this period, the "signs" continued to abound. Some of them were so profound that, to this day, they carry a personal significance bordering on the spiritual. (In fact, some people who disagree with the medical view of "mental illness" – even some cultures – suggest that the symptoms I experienced are really a state of heightened consciousness. A perspective that, though appealing, doesn't really explain why I'd blow all my money or sabotage the career I'd worked years to advance.)

Yet many of these signs were quite striking. Consider what happened when I purchased, during a trip to the market, a button with the Chinese character for "dragon" written on it.

A dragon, of course, is a powerful icon in Chinese culture. I figured this might just be a powerful button and pinned it to my shirt. The next day, we took a trip to the Great Wall, stopping at a tourist store en route. Inside was a woman – a master carver of small Chinese gourds – selling her work. I was drawn to one immediately; it depicted two dragons in struggle over a flaming pearl.

This particular image is omnipresent in China, one which can be interpreted in many ways: the balance between heaven and earth, between man and woman, between good and evil. I believed both the button and the gourd had potent, mystical powers.

As we climbed the Great Wall, we came upon many vendors selling similar buttons. I searched in vain to find another dragon button for Julia, convinced that, for the balance to be complete, I *had to* obtain one for her.

But no one had the same button – until we reached the highest point of the wall. A seller there thought he might have one left and started looking through bags and bags of his stock. He sorted through a jumble of many hundreds of buttons.

The more he looked, the more intent I was that I find another dragon. Just as he was about to tell me he had none, he found one. It was at the bottom of the very last bag.

Unlike all the other buttons, it was not new. It was old, dirty, scratched. It had the look of a clever prop in a Spielberg movie, something that was supposed to look inherently evil. As he dropped it in my palm, there was a loud and disturbing *crack* behind me.

I turned to see a man with blood pouring from his forehead.

There was a second *crack* as a man struck him again with a lead pipe.

A mob began to beat the injured man furiously (I never learned why) and nearly threw him over the wall. This was not my imagination. Julia, horrified, witnessed it as well. And it was the only extreme violence – with the exception of Tiananmen – that I'd ever witnessed in China.

All this transpired in seconds. And it began at the precise instant that the button touched my flesh. When you've got sprouting delusions, believe me, this was not a good thing to have witnessed.

There were *many* such coincidences. In some feedback loop of the psyche, they were both indicators of the disorder – and fuel for it.

On the anniversary of the Chinese army's move into Tiananmen Square, a furious storm hit Beijing. We stared in wonder from our hotel window, and I videotaped, as a Chinese construction crew trapped on a crane screamed for their lives. The crane was swaying so heavily in the winds, we were sure it would topple.

I was thinking, at that moment, how the Chinese often interpret such storms or natural disasters as signs that the heavens are displeased with their rulers – that the so-called "Mandate of Heaven" granting leadership is about to expire. And this, as I knew, was the anniversary of Tiananmen Square.

At that moment, a lightning bolt struck and set fire to an electrical substation outside our window, sending a fury of blue sparks sizzling through the air.

You get the picture.

So imagine. The secrets of the universe are revealing themselves to you. You have been *chosen* to receive this knowledge. You are here for a *reason*. Deep stuff.

I was now convinced that I had indeed been selected by a higher power. My task was to battle the forces of evil, as exemplified by that beat-up old dragon button.

As this delusion progressed, my emotions became highly volatile. Normally, I hold my cards pretty close to my chest. Now, however, joy and compassion flooded my veins. I recall meeting a severely disabled beggar on the street, a man missing his legs and both eyes. I sat, held his hand, stared into those dark, empty sockets. I then gently gave him a large amount of currency and told him to get something good to eat and drink. He reached out and embraced me with a warmth that seemed to come directly from God. I wept, humbled.

Conversely, I could explode in anger in an instant. While visiting the Ming tombs not far from the wall, a money-changer tried to cheat me out of $100 U.S. In a flash I grabbed him by his shirt collar and let loose a torrent of Chinese profanity. My anger was so intense I was almost looking for an excuse to hit him. Instead, he quickly returned the money, and the moment he did so, I was calm. Explosions like that are completely foreign to me; I haven't been in a fight since high school.

Poor Julia, meanwhile, was trapped. Stuck in a country she didn't know, with a language she didn't know, with a man she didn't know.

She tried repeatedly, desperately – even frantically – to point out her concerns. But even when she listed the symptoms, even when the evidence was right there in front of me, I could not see the problem. Quite the opposite. The problem, if there was one, was with *Julia* for not appreciating the tremendous and positive transformation I had undergone. There was nothing wrong with me; on the contrary, I was becoming more enlightened with every footstep. I was not merely a Buddhist, I was one of the coolest Buddhists ever. Felt like I was walking on air.

And I was still going up.

At the airport for the flight back to Hong Kong, we discovered that our video camera, which I'd used to document much of my spiritual transformation, was missing. After reporting the loss, we got on board. An elderly Tibetan monk, robes flowing, was sitting two rows in front of us. He would know, I thought, where the camera was, how to get it back. *He would know.*

I sat in a contemplative state, waiting for some sign that I should contact him. The answer came, calmly, in a single word. "Yes." An actual voice, resolute, compelling, filled my head. "*Yes.*" Except no one near me was speaking.

One might think, given that I'd never heard a voice in my head during the previous thirty-four years of my life, that I might find this odd. Instead, it was exhilarating. I had, I believed, achieved a state of telepathy – a notion confirmed when I glanced at the woman sitting across the aisle. She appeared to be, was clearly, in a meditative trance. Sending thoughtful Buddhist messages directly into my receptive little Buddhist head. (I now suspect she was merely asleep.)

I walked over to the monk, handed him the small carved gourd and my Amex gold card, which I believed would aid his mystical powers. He accepted the items and closed his eyes. He would, I knew, use those powers to find our camera. We never did recover it. (Julia, however, managed to retrieve the credit card.)

By the time we reached Hong Kong, I had completely broken with reality. I was in my *own* reality. Everything I'm about to describe actually happened. What I saw, you would have seen. But it was the *way* I saw it, the way I interpreted these messages, that was different.

As I stood at the edge of the harbour, something told me to drop my running shoes into the water.

Plop. Plop.

They began to float, right-side up, toward the ocean. They remained parallel, though the right, then the left, would advance in turn. They were, it appeared, walking on water. I bathed my feet in a puddle and turned. The word "wise" was hand-painted on scores of huge wooden spools in a storage yard. I was wise.

Four crates, which looked like coffins, were stacked near the water. Three of them were labelled "CH," which I believed referred to the three occasions I was in danger in Chechnya. The fourth was labelled "SS," my initials. This was powerful stuff. I noticed a long staff of bamboo beside me. Exact dimensions of a fishing pole. I picked it up and began to walk, barefoot.

I felt like Christ. Buddha.

Both.

We reached a hotel where, once inside our room, I set up a Buddhist spirit house purchased in Beijing. I lit a candle and surrounded the house with all manner of artifacts from the trip, including a Buddha, three original paintings, and a solid gold watch given to me by one of China's most prominent artists. With the proper placement of the objects, the right ritual, I believed the battle against evil would be won.

The entire room became a mystical jigsaw puzzle as I rearranged items to focus the energy of the universe. A candle here, a Buddha there. . . . I was intent on performing this little cosmic shuffle until a sign came that the battle had been won. Julia was truly frightened. (Not an unreasonable reaction. I mean, face it, I was *nuts*.)

At one point I stood motionless on one leg on top of a chair, a pose that may or may not have had its roots in Tai Qi. I tried to cleanse Julia's fear, her inability to see the world through my reborn eyes, by splashing Chinese liquor on her – the equivalent, in my state of mind, of holy water. I even threw the three paintings, worth thousands of dollars and much more on a personal level, out the window as an offering to the gods. The gods never came.

But in the morning, thanks to Julia, an ambulance did.

I had not slept all night, was still trying to trigger the Second Coming, when the attendants arrived. I had actually filled the bathtub with sacred objects and was baptizing myself when they came into the room. When I met them – soaking wet and half naked – I explained there was no problem, only that I couldn't sleep, that I was filled with *Qi*, or energy.

"What kind of *Qi*?" asked the paramedic. "*This kind*," I said, assuming a martial-arts stance and effortlessly punching a neat hole through the closet door.

The paramedic, to his great credit, worked *with* the psychosis instead of against it. He did not restrain me, did not threaten force. Instead, he calmly put his hands together and began to chant a Buddhist prayer for peace. *Ahhh*, I thought, *a fellow Buddhist. Someone good. Perhaps it is time to . . . rest.* I lay down on the bed, felt myself begin to relax, and allowed myself to be placed on a stretcher. It was the first time in weeks I'd felt a semblance of calm. It was blissful.

Slowly, gently, they tied me down with strips of cloth. There was no coercion; they could not have handled the situation more sensitively.

Yet soon after reaching the hospital, I was again feeling energized. Enough resting. This hospital thing was surely part of my mission, my *test*. I asked a doctor if I was free to leave; he said I was. I wandered the hospital halls, dressed only in a gown, followed by police. I kept noticing signs with arrows pointing toward the morgue. I interpreted these as omens, that the hospital equalled mortal danger. I had to get out of there.

As I was taking my stroll, the doctor was filling in the paperwork to have me involuntarily hospitalized. He notified the officers.

Just outside the hospital, I found my way onto a small commuter train. The police ordered the driver not to continue on his route. I screamed to the passengers, "If any of you are Buddhists, *please* help me!" I then grabbed the overhead pole and mentally welded my hands in place. I pictured myself as a tree, an oak that could not be budged.

It took five officers some time before I *was* budged. They handcuffed me with such force they cut one wrist. I was in absolute terror as they dragged me back into the hospital. (Where were those nice Buddhist ambulance guys when I needed them?) An orderly and nurses came running toward me. I believed I was about to die.

With the police assisting, they pinned me to a bed. I continued struggling as a large syringe was plunged deep into my thigh.

I was screaming when I passed out.

After the injection wore off – which took only twenty minutes, despite the staff telling Julia I'd be out for hours – I awoke to find myself thoroughly restrained. Not just by a straitjacket, but by long strips of cloth tightly binding my ankles and wrists to the bed. Trust me, the Chinese tie excellent knots.

Still manic, I was determined to escape. "Why did you let them tie me up?" I asked Julia. "I was finally free." Julia did her best to reassure me, told me I was in a place where people were trying to help me. Though tearful, she was remarkably calm – a deep and quiet strength she would demonstrate in abundance in the months ahead.

I no longer believed I would die if I remained in the hospital, but getting out of the straitjacket – gaining freedom from restraint – seemed the most important mission on earth.

Slowly, with remarkable agility for a single bound hand, I began to manipulate the knots crushing my right wrist.

One knot came undone, then another. My left hand began to pluck toward its own freedom. Soon, the tight cluster of knots was gone. I even managed, in a manoeuvre worthy of Houdini, to remove the straitjacket itself, much to the astonishment of hospital staff.

"YOU!" screamed a huge orderly. "You . . . sit . . . STILL!" he boomed.

I did, in a cross-legged pose befitting my exalted Buddhist stature.

I was taken to a massive crumbling complex just outside the city (again tied up for the ambulance run) and kept there on a judge's order for five days. I was the only Caucasian, and, with the exception of the doctors, few patients spoke English. To speak with them, I had to rely on my Mandarin.

"Why are you here?" asked a fellow patient.

"I have too much Qi," I explained.

"I also have too much Qi," he replied. "I bit my sister."

Delusions are adaptable things, highly malleable to situation. That I was locked up against my will did not occur to me. That I was surrounded by people in varying degrees of psychosis did not trouble me. I believed, as the ambulance attendant had told me, I was going to "a nice place." A place where devout Buddhists like myself were meant to gather, to use our powers collectively. In a matter of days, I thought, we would be changing the world. War, poverty, inequity would end – all thanks to our impending Buddhist brainstorm.

On arrival, I was segregated, along with five other patients, from the general population of the ward. It was night, and most of the others were in a smoking area enclosed by a chain-link fence outside our sole window. I could make out only dark shadows, the faint glint of eyes, as they stared in at the new arrival. Perhaps they were evil, perhaps my job was to convert them. I held a cigarette to the window as an initial peace offering. A quick movement plucked the smoke from my hand; a moment later a freshly lit cigarette was offered back. Progress.

The clinical staff was fascinated to have a Western journalist in their midst. Surprised, too. They told me the same ward had been the involuntary home to a major U.S. network correspondent the previous week. He had scrawled his well-known name on the wall. One nurse was particularly intrigued by the fact that I had recently been in Moscow, Chechnya, Beijing, and now Hong Kong. Also that I could speak passable Mandarin. "Are you a spy?" he asked me repeatedly. "You must be a spy. Are you a spy?" (Excellent therapy for a delusional man locked up in a foreign asylum.)

The staff could not initially reach a diagnosis. Although they suspected a mood disorder, they told Julia that hearing a voice is often a symptom of schizophrenia. We would both learn that the diagnosis of mental disorder is far from a pure science.

The picture became clearer when I kept talking (a lot) about all the Qi I had. So much Qi that even strong sedatives did not put me to sleep at night. Plus, I was so damn cheerful, despite being locked up. The staff eventually settled on bipolar affective disorder. Can't say it meant much to me at the time. I still figured I was on some heavenly mission – a delusion if ever there was one, given the conditions I was housed in.

I have many memories of that facility, of the caged fences, the locks, the filth. But those that endure involve the kindness shown by fellow patients. The sharing of food. Of cigarettes. Of situation. One older Chinese man, with an empathy and compassion I shall always remember, helped undress and shower me in a small washroom. Despite the excrement fouling the floor, there was a remarkable dignity to the act.

While I was nuts on the inside, Julia was going nuts on the outside. Trying to cope with the fact that her partner was in a psychiatric hospital. Trying to keep family members up to date with the situation. Trying to figure out how to get me out of there and back home. Trying to cope with almost all of this on her own, halfway around the world.

Close friends and colleagues – including Peter Mansbridge – called each of us in Hong Kong to offer assistance. Mansbridge sagely reminded me that I was blessed with a remarkable woman. A good pal, Tom, gave Julia his calling-card number and told her to make as many overseas calls as she liked. (It was the first of his many acts of kindness during this nightmare. Neither of us will ever forget that support.)

Yet not a single editorial manager – people I'd worked with for years and considered my friends – called Julia to ask how I was. And that, too, is something I shall never forget – and still struggle to comprehend.

It was in stark contrast to other situations where CBC employees have been ill while abroad. In one case, a correspondent was hit by a rubber bullet in the West Bank. A manager flew from London to ensure he received the best possible care. Another employee, with an alcohol-abuse problem, had been directed to treatment.

But there's something about a *mental* disorder that changes all the rules. The standard responses to physical illnesses go out the window. There is an awkwardness, a fear, a silence. People don't know how to react. I've since met many other people, from many other fields, who've had similar experiences.

After several calls, Julia found out that my insurance would cover a flight back to Canada. In the company of a nurse, we flew from Hong Kong back to Vancouver, where my father met us, and then on to Saskatoon, my hometown. I was, though now on medication, still in outer space. And in a remarkably good mood, considering I'd blown both my bank account and my career. Believe it or not, I was also still spending. I nearly ordered a $3,000 hot tub for our cabin.

We went to the hospital for another assessment. While sitting in the waiting room, I noticed a wheelchair with "PSYCHIATRY" stencilled on the back. I pointed it out to my mother, chuckling. Despite everything I'd been through, I was still convinced that I was in perfect health, that the real problem was the failure of others to recognize that something extraordinary and wonderful had happened to me. That I had been spiritually reborn. That my limitless potential had finally been freed.

So my family was faced with a difficult task. Doctors told them it would be best if they could convince me to accept hospitalization; another involuntary committal might not be productive. The doctor was convinced, rightly, that I would freak out if a bunch of people grabbed me again. There was also the fact that I only barely met the legal criteria in Saskatchewan to be held against my will.

We had, over the course of days, several meetings with that doctor at University Hospital. Eventually, more to please my family than anything else, I accepted voluntary hospitalization. Staff asked me, on admission, if I had any "sharps." Huh? "You know, sharp things. Razor, knife, scissors?" I handed over my razor, still not knowing why they wanted it (at the time, harming myself was the furthest thing from my mind). Only one friend sent flowers; they arrived in a cardboard container, because all glass is banned from the ward.

They continued me on the antipsychotic drug I'd been given in Hong Kong: haloperidol, "Haldol" for short. They also put me on lithium, a common treatment for this disorder. After about two weeks, the drugs started dragging the mania – and all joy – out of me. I felt like crap. And was finally starting to realize what had happened.

We returned to Toronto, where the Haldol continued to transform me into a slug. I walked like an old man – nurses call it "The Haldol Shuffle" – and felt like one. A new doctor, whom it took weeks to find and for whom I had to wait further weeks to see, spent about ten minutes with me and wrote out a prescription for several drugs. He told me to come back in a few months. The medications caused my vision to blur to the point where I could not read. My skin broke out in spots. I had been warned of *none* of these side effects – nor of Haldol's potential to cause tardive dyskinesia, a sometimes permanent disorder that can cause involuntary facial grimaces.

The medication deemed necessary to save me felt like it would kill me. I would later learn that at one point the amount of Haldol I was being given was many times the recommended therapeutic dose. It's small wonder I felt so awful. Though I am not anti-medication, I can understand why some people are. The Buddhist quickly gave way to the zombie. I felt like I was aging, withering. Disintegrating.

We were invited, a few weeks later, to a brunch to celebrate a friend's marriage. I attended, in such a fog of drugs I felt trapped in another dimension. I recall a profound sense of shame that day, an awareness that previously close friends were avoiding eye contact. I felt a desperate, helpless need to somehow explain that this shuffling shell, this stranger with the slow speech and the dead eyes, was not me. But I was so ashamed, deeply ashamed, I could not speak those words. Nor did I believe anyone could possibly understand what I meant by them.

The reality of my situation was beginning to sink in.

And then, of course, the furniture arrived. An entire container load.

The spiral into depression was fast. Part of that depression is the natural cycle of the disorder: what goes up, must come down. But a large part of it was situational. There was, of course, the pure shock of having been diagnosed with a serious mental disorder, a label I feared would curse me forever. But there were more tangible problems, lots of them.

I'd lost what I'd coveted most during my professional career: a foreign posting. I'd spent all my money. My reputation was toast.

And we had all that cursed furniture. So much that what didn't fit in a rented storage facility filled our condo to the ceiling. Aside from Julia, it was the last thing I saw each night, the first thing I saw each morning. What seemed like all the furniture in China. Believe me, that combination of circumstances would make *anyone* depressed.

The road to recovery was a long one.

I spent weeks in bed, unable to find any reason to get up. Sleep was my drug – the only, albeit temporary, way to escape what had befallen me. When awake I brooded, almost obsessively, on death. Pictured myself rigging pulleys so I could hang myself in the condo, figured with *two* pulleys I could actually haul myself up. Browsed through *Final Exit*, a suicide manual, while in a bookstore.

Deep down, I knew I would not kill myself, knew it would cause others too much pain. But the tantalizing *thought* of it – what's known as "suicidal ideation" – filled my head almost constantly. Most mornings, the first thought that entered my head was to put a gun to it. *Bang*. Problem solved.

When not thinking of death, my only diversion was to wistfully fantasize that it had been a physical injury; I wished countless times for a horrendous war wound instead. If only a bullet had shattered my arm, a mortar blown off my leg. That, I could come to terms with. Anything but *this*.

In September, all our personal belongings from Moscow arrived back in Toronto. An immutable reminder of all that had been lost. I knew that to be in the house that day would be more than I could bear.

Julia, perceptive as always, insisted I go for a walk and practically pushed me out the door. I did, postponing my return for as long as possible. In fact, I didn't want to go back at all, dreading what I would find. But I had little choice. The condo was filled again, this time with boxes from the place where it all began, a cardboard monument to madness and failure. I was inconsolable.

Just then the phone rang. It was my former manager. He explained that my mother had called him, told him what terrible shape I was in. He sounded genuinely concerned, much like the person I remembered pre-crisis. I was sobbing, trying to sound composed, wiping snot from my nose and tears from my cheeks, feeling totally crushed. Feeling ashamed, too, that I sounded so hopelessly *weak*. That's when he said he'd like to come over and talk.

"You have no idea," I choked, "what that would mean to me." He said he couldn't come that day, but I'd see him soon. I felt hope for the first time since this nightmare began.

He never called back.

My purpose in writing this isn't to blame anyone. In all honesty, I'm not sure what *I* would have done in his shoes. Psychological pain is not an easy thing to deal with – and I was in definite pain. I should also say that the CBC, in all other bureaucratic aspects, did everything right. There was good long-term disability insurance, my medication was paid for, a job was still there. All of that stuff was done to the letter.

But the silence which followed that phone call plunged me into greater despair. Part of it was the disorder itself – I was already in a deep depression – but there's an ingredient to recovery that, I believe, is at least as important as the chemicals I was ingesting. *Hope.* The belief that you're still worth something after an episode like this, that the people who recognized your skills in the past will recognize those skills still exist. That a bout with a mental disorder does not mean you have *become* the disorder. That life can go on.

Later that month we managed, with considerable difficulty, and through the connections of a friend, to locate another psychiatrist. Julia came to the first session and did most of the talking. I remember being able to utter only two desperate words that day: "Help me." And this physician did. I got the sense she cared about my situation, that she viewed me as an individual beyond the diagnosis. She was careful to lay out for me the benefits and risks of all medication – and was respectful of my eventual decision to try living without them. She listened, with genuine sympathy and concrete advice, when I explained (over and over again) how crushed I was over everything that had happened. Ultimately, however, she was only one component – albeit an important one – in a far greater system of care crucial to my return to wellness.

The foundation of which was Julia. She suffered every bit as deeply as I did during this odyssey, sacrificing much along the way. It would have been so easy, so understandable, for her simply to walk away from all this. But she did not.

My family, too, helped share the awful burden. They called often, enduring the relentless misery they heard in my voice. It was not easy for them to hear such chronic agony, but they persisted. A small – then smaller – core of friends showed tremendous understanding and patience. At the time, these were thankless tasks. But they were important ones. Our tendency is to shun people with mental health difficulties. To leave them alone until they get over it.

Almost no one gets over it alone.

My good friend Tom called nearly every night, even when my only news was that I'd figured out a new method of suicide. My neighbour and pal Dave kept inviting me over for movies, even when I didn't laugh during comedies. Both included me in a trip to Chicago where, appropriately enough, we went to blues clubs.

My chum Daryl flew from Saskatoon to visit me at the cabin during that first, awful summer back in Canada. He didn't pressure me to snap out of it, force me to go canoeing when I wanted to retreat to bed at noon. He listened when I felt like talking, amused himself when I didn't. My cousin Drew sent flowers when he heard the story, then took me out for lunch and offered some advice for dealing with the dreaded furniture. Dianne, who helped sell the furniture at her Toronto store, encouraged me to come over and visit at length – a welcome respite from yet another day of staring at the ceiling. Our new friend David never failed to invite us to his social gatherings, even when I couldn't appreciate his wit.

One day during that extended black hole, Al (the Estonian!) came over to visit. He offered a very simple truth.

"You're sick now, buddy," he said. "But you won't always be."

He was right. (And every one of those people, God bless them, bought some furniture!)

The contribution of *all* these people and others to my recovery can never be overestimated: I simply would not have made it without them. And certainly not without Julia. How she managed to cope, for *months*, is a study in courage, giving, love.

And in persistence.

She found me one fall afternoon when the depression reached its blackest. Zero light. I was lying around in my bathrobe, despite the late hour. This was not unusual. What was unusual was that I had pretty much given up. It's difficult to articulate, but it felt as though my will had simply surrendered. A tattered white flag flapping dimly in the shadows. My life, as I knew it, was over. Finished.

And, as usual, I had not eaten.

Julia heated soup. Chicken noodle. But comfort food cannot comfort someone who feels only dread. I had neither the strength nor the desire to lift the spoon to my lips. There was just no reason to. No point. So Julia did it for me.

Tears began to well. I could feel her love, knew what a beautiful act this was. But I felt dead inside, wanted only for this agony to end. At thirty-five years of age, a man who once had a promising career, I felt more helpless than an infant.

Julia called my doctor, who recommended voluntary hospitalization. Reluctantly, I accepted her advice and checked in to Toronto's Mount Sinai Hospital the following morning. I stayed there at night, but was free to leave during the day. It was at that time perhaps an appropriate place for me. We did not know that there are alternatives for people in crisis; it seemed hospital was the only option.

The treatment was a combination of talk therapy, blood tests to determine if something else was contributing to the depression, and medication adjustment. I held out little hope that changing the dose of antidepressants would make me feel much better. But the talk therapy did help. I connected with another caring, listening psychiatrist at the hospital; a professional who gave me some hope. Yet unloading the furniture – and rebuilding a career – still seemed impossible. (By this time, we had moved the furniture to a warehouse, from which we hoped to sell it. I had to force myself to go there, so abundant was the evidence of my madness. I absolutely dripped with gloom; a mortician would have made a better salesman.)

Despite my bleak state of mind at Mount Sinai, there were a couple of moments that triggered the faint echo of a smile. Like smoking in the washroom after the nurse had made her rounds, balancing carefully on the toilet while blowing into the exhaust fan. The bathroom was much cleaner than in Hong Kong. There were also people there (though I hate these kinds of comparisons) in much worse shape than me.

The antidepressants did, eventually, give me enough of a boost that I was better able to start tackling the furniture – with tremendous help from Julia. And also from my father, Lyle, who flew to Toronto to offer support and help assemble the blasted opium beds. There were three of them, each with a multitude of fiendishly clever interlocking pieces – and no instructions. I was not able to give my dad much assistance, but he kept at it. And, more importantly, *listened* to me when I tried to articulate the hell I was enduring.

That was as important to me as any drug I received.

Over time, a long time, I began to realize I would survive. The remaining furniture wound up in Dianne's store and slowly diminished. The medication was, again, reduced. And gradually, finally, the blessed markers of normal life began to creep back in.

Food started to regain its taste. There became reasons to shave. One day, without even realizing it, I remembered how to smile. One night, gazing toward a crimson skyline, I relearned that a sunset is more than a prelude to night.

Though it felt like forever, I *did* recover – enough that my psychiatrist recommended to the CBC that I be returned to a foreign posting. Indeed, she felt it was crucial to my mental health that I go back to a job as challenging as my old one. I met with my new manager and said I'd like to return to Moscow.

"That's impossible," I was told. When I asked why, the response was repeated. "That's just impossible."

I've wondered, since then, what my response would have been if the roles were reversed. I honestly don't know. We eventually agreed on a producing position for *Midday News*.

Returning to a job of lower stature was a demeaning experience, a daily reminder of what had been lost. I was also completely out of the loop I'd once been part of – those whose editorial opinions are sought out and valued. And that was the least of it.

Most colleagues said a polite "hello" and little else. Some didn't even say hi, preferring instead to avert their eyes to some invisible distraction on the floor.

It's just my imagination, I thought. Except it wasn't. People *did* look at me differently, regard me differently, treat me differently. (Some colleagues – Havard, Susan, Marc, and others – were great. Unfortunately, they were the exceptions.)

Dismayed, I sought the advice of a couple of senior people I trusted. One offered this uplifting bit of advice: "You were lucky," he said, "they didn't fire you." The other said simply, "In the space of one day your reputation, in the minds of many, went from being very high to rock bottom."

So I learned a thing or too about stigma along the way. Discovered that it can be more painful than the disorder itself. Realized that some people, perhaps many, still cling to the view that mental disorder is an indication of personal weakness.

Or maybe they're just plain scared of it. Scores of people have since told me about what happened to them in their workplaces, and it's clear my experience was not unique.

One of the hardest things was learning from two top specialists that if the disorder had been caught during its early phase in Moscow, I could have been treated and back at work within two weeks. But that's a very big "if," given that neither of us was aware of what we were dealing with.

Throughout it all – the diagnosis, the depression, the drugs – I struggled to find some shred of meaning in what had happened to me. I am not a deeply religious or spiritual person, but I do believe in a certain balance in life. And I needed, very much, to find the answer to a single question: *What purpose did this serve?*

The answer came on February 20, 1997, when Edmond Yu, a homeless Chinese man with a diagnosis of paranoid schizophrenia, was shot to death by Toronto police. Edmond, a Hong Kong immigrant, was killed while cornered on a bus. I could not ignore the parallel, and thought immediately of my own terrifying minutes confronting police in the city of his birth.

His death challenged me to try to take two tragedies – Edmond's and my own – and turn them into something meaningful. As a journalist, as a human being, I wanted to know more about his life, the circumstances that had led him to that bus that fateful day.

I applied for, and received, an Atkinson Fellowship in Public Policy. The award, granted to one Canadian journalist annually by the Atkinson Charitable Foundation in Toronto, allows for a year of investigative research into an area of compelling public policy. The selection committee decided my topic had merit: mental health.

That year, 1997–98, was a voyage of discovery. It led to a week-long series of articles in the *Toronto Star* called "Out of Mind." The first story in that series was a condensed version of what you are reading now. The story of Edmond Yu also appeared the same day, and many have said it forever altered how they perceive the homeless with mental disorders. (You can find that story at <http://atkinsonfdn.on.ca/>. Click on "Publications" then on "Out of Mind.")

The day those stories came out the headline read: "MY INCREDIBLE VOYAGE INTO MADNESS – AND BACK." I literally choked when I saw my words and photo there on the front page. I wondered if I had done the right thing, if it was worth taking this personal risk.

And then the phone started to ring. Calls of congratulations from both friends and strangers. Calls from people in similar situations, asking for advice. And, pleasantly, calls from some senior news folk at the CBC. They wanted to pass along their best wishes, and tell me they understood why I had written the story.

Those calls, and many more, helped restore a self-esteem that had been tested to the very limits. The work led to numerous awards and was part of a combined entry that earned the *Star* a Michener Award, one of the highest journalism honours in Canada.

It also led to a new job. Just as the Atkinson Charitable Foundation had viewed my fellowship proposal based on its own merits, so too was I judged by the *Star*. I was not viewed as a "manic-depressive," but as a journalist (though I've since learned from some colleagues that the two are by no means mutually exclusive). In short, a career I believed was over has, in many ways, just begun.

Nearly a year after joining the *Star*, I received an assignment that was a turning point for me. It began when I was working late one Friday and my boss emerged from a meeting.

"Got a valid passport?" he asked.

"Yes."

"How do you feel about going to Ethiopia?"

Many journalists, at such a question, would be thrilled at the offer. Instead, my heart sank so deep I swear it fell out of my left pant leg.

"Umm, fine," I said with a weak smile.

In truth, I was terrified. The last time I'd been someplace hard and far away was Chechnya – and we all know how *that* turned out. Yet part of me wanted to test myself, to see if it was possible to work on a tough and miserable story, a famine, without my mental health failing. Another part was tremendously grateful that the *Star*, knowing my history, would be willing to take a chance on this trip. I didn't want to disappoint the newspaper, nor myself. After discussing it with Julia, and with my psychiatrist, I decided to go.

Two days before departure, I dropped into the office of a senior manager I trusted.

"I'm really pleased that you considered me for this trip," I told him. "But I'm also a bit nervous. There was that thing in Chechnya, you know."

"Yes," he replied with a chuckle. "That did dawn on me." He then pulled out a piece of paper, on which he wrote two phone numbers.

"This is my home number, this is my cell. If anything starts happening, at any time, and you feel like you need to call, no problem. Day or night."

"Don't worry," he added. "This trip will be good for you."

That simple gesture was incredibly important. I arrived in Ethiopia knowing there was support back home: from my employer, from Julia, my family, and my doctor (who'd also given me a home number and all the appropriate medications, just in case).

It was, of course, a difficult trip. So severe was the drought that the country's south was a desert of suffering. Untold numbers of fresh graves dotted the roadside; trails of dust littered with the bones and hides of desiccated animals. It was a desolate and depressing place.

But I watched myself. Made sure I got a reasonably decent sleep every night (not an easy task in a rural Ethiopian brothel!), avoided the mistakes I'd made in Moscow, and stayed focused on the job. The first story got filed, then the next, then the next. I did not need to make that phone call to my boss. And I knew, upon my return, that I was capable of taking such a trip again.

In some ways, I've been one of the lucky ones. I have been able, with the co-operation and respect of a good doctor, to manage this thing without the constant use of medications. I have used them when necessary, and would take them again if required. But I have also taken other steps to ensure my stability.

Certainly I've made changes in lifestyle, with more to come. I make sure I keep regular hours, try to eat well, and don't party like I used to. I know, as does Julia and my family, what the warning signs are. Something's up, literally, if I get a sudden urge to fly to China and buy furniture. (Which, mercifully, has not happened.) When I feel medication is necessary, I take it. When I can manage things on my own, which is the vast majority of the time, I do. I'm taking a certain risk here, but so far so good.

Many others diagnosed with bipolar affective disorder have not been so fortunate. Some people literally owe their stability to the proper meds, and I am in no way suggesting that my experience is typical or some model to emulate. There is always the chance that I may again dip down or start soaring. It is a risk I have chosen to take, based both on being informed about the benefits and drawbacks of medication, and – perhaps more than anything – on getting to know myself. I've still got some work to do in that area. But so do we all.

You may well assume that after having survived the twin nightmares of mania and depression, I would do anything to go back in time – to have nipped it in the bud. It's a reasonable assumption. And an impossibility I once obsessively longed for. Not just for myself. But for Julia. My family. My friends.

After much reflection, I have learned how futile – destructive even – that retrospective angst can be. Over time, I have finally accepted what took place. It's taken some doing, but I've managed to let go of the bitterness, the anger, the grief.

Madness, though destructive, has also been *instructive*.

It allowed me to explore – and survive – the very extremes of human experience.

I have known what it is like to feel like a God. And I've known what it is like to be condemned to hell. Things a relatively small number of people will ever know – at least in this lifetime.

I certainly would not wish it on anyone else.

But I have *been* those two Chinese dragons.

I have learned from them.

And – with help – survived them.

CHAPTER TWO

Julia's Story

By the time we left for Moscow, I figured I'd seen it all. Maybe every twenty-nine-year-old thinks that way. But in my own mind, I was different. I'd lived in Ottawa, Montreal, Toronto, Vancouver, London, and Prague. I'd been a newspaper writer, a TV reporter, a radio producer.

And in those jobs, I'd written on any number of topics. Even health-related ones. I had sat, one grey and tear-filled afternoon, in the home of a couple whose baby had just died of meningitis. I had visited a chemotherapy ward, interviewing a young woman about breast cancer while the steady drip of chemicals entered her body.

We journalists grow accustomed to such exposure. The tragedies we've seen, the sorrows we've witnessed; they touch us, but not directly. We get used to bad things happening to *other* people.

And then I went to Moscow with Scott. And I learned what tragedy and sorrow feel like first-hand, close-up, deep within myself. Also, I learned just how little I knew. On the subject of *mental* health, I was woefully uninformed. I'd never written about mental disorder, never knowingly spoken with anyone who had one.

Six years later, I still feel like the fool. The person who should have known but didn't. Could have seen, intervened, acted sooner, but somehow wouldn't. I think that anyone reading Scott's story must inevitably think me daft.

What's helped me most is talking to other people. I've learned that, on this one topic, ignorance is commonplace. Who thinks about depression, mania, or mental distress unless it stares them in the face? Who knows the warning signs, the symptoms, the look or sound of madness until it strikes in their own home?

Whether it's meningitis or mood disorder, people share their stories for two reasons. They want people in the same situation to know they're not alone. And they want anyone who isn't – who has not seen what they've seen or survived what they have – to stand forewarned and take precautions.

As a journalist, I came to understand this. Now I'm doing the same, sharing my story for those same two reasons.

I remember the mixed reactions when I told people we were moving to Russia. Some people were enthusiastic. "How exciting!" they said. "How romantic!" Others were perplexed. "Why the hell would you go *there*?" they asked.

Anyone who *has* been there will tell you, Moscow is not an easy place to live. No wonder the Russians are renowned for their sturdiness. Chronically grey skies, sporadic hot water, push-and-shove sidewalks, lung-blackening pollution: this was what greeted us in Moscow. A head of lettuce could cost several dollars and sending a fax could take an entire afternoon. It took some getting used to.

In September, I wrote in my journal: *Tanya [our language tutor] told us foreigners must escape at least once every three months or they go crazy. And I'm starting to understand why. "What about Russians?" I asked. "They go crazy too," she said. "But they have no choice."*

Those first few months, Scott seemed to be especially down on the place. We both complained – all expats do – but Scott seemed less willing to keep trying, get to know the city, find the good stuff about it. Sometimes, he even said he wished he hadn't come.

His negativity was surprising; Scott had travelled widely and lived abroad before. Surely he knew it wouldn't be easy. I couldn't understand why he was letting the city get to him so. But get to him it did. That fall, I watched Scott's mood slip. And I responded by trying to cheer him up.

I remember one Sunday walk in a park, a rare escape from the interminable noise and traffic of the city centre. The last of the leaves had fallen, and the crunching sound underfoot was familiar, like home. Ducks floated serenely on a shallow pond and the air seemed miraculously clean. Caught up in the moment, I grabbed a handful of dry leaves and, giggling, dumped them onto Scott's head. I stood there waiting for him to respond. But he didn't laugh. Didn't even crack a smile. He just kept walking, shoulders hunched, the leaves falling away.

What's *wrong* with him? I thought.

Depression, I now know, has a certain look. But in those early days I did not recognize it. Scott's eyes had grown dull, his movements slow, his shoulders forever slouched forward. He seemed always to be thinking of something else, even as I spoke to him.

Other people noticed too, and commented.

October 26: *A cold, grey, rainy Wednesday. . . . "Now you know why Russians like to drink so much," said Tanya. She was trying to get a laugh out of Scott – shocked to see his face after several weeks without lessons. "He looks absolutely miserable," she said when she saw him. "Julia, shto delat?" (What to do?) She wasn't exaggerating. It's true. He is miserable.*

What to do, indeed? I knew Scott had been through a mild depression once before. But I hadn't witnessed it first-hand; we were only friends then, living in separate cities. He'd travelled to Thailand, his mood had plummeted, and his doctor had recommended an antidepressant. Before we left for

Moscow, Scott had stopped taking the pills. I hadn't thought much about it at the time; he seemed so patently well. But was the same thing happening again?

We talked about another prescription, a doctor's visit, perhaps some psychotherapy. In Canada, he might have tried these things; I might have pushed for them harder. But in Moscow we had no family doctor to call upon, no English-speaking psychiatrist close at hand. It seemed easier, somehow, just to keep plodding on.

Besides, it was easy to believe Scott wasn't actually ill. He was getting up every morning, working long hours, eating and sleeping, even partying occasionally with new friends. He was just unhappy, and in time convinced that Moscow was the reason why.

December 5: *Scott left for the office, depressed as usual. . . . [He] has been consumed of late with getting the hell out of here. . . . Every morning, he drags himself out of bed, face grim, shoulders slouched, recovering from yet another bad dream . . .*

By the New Year, Scott had become unhappy with everything: the job, the city, even his relationship with me. Doubt plagued him; surely one or all of these things accounted for his misery. He talked about moving back to Canada, staying in Moscow but changing jobs, or breaking up with me. I think the only thing that stopped him from taking these steps was a certain guilt about how I'd be affected.

As Scott's despair grew, so did the precariousness of my own situation. For the first time in my adult life, I was partially dependent. Barely settled in Moscow, living in an apartment paid for by Scott's employer, I had no full-time job. (I had quit my CBC job in Canada to come here and had only just begun freelance work.) So I listened to Scott's complaints with a growing sense of panic. I mean, he was talking about *dumping* me.

I did my best to be supportive. Empathized, listened, made suggestions. But none of that helped. And so my frustration grew. With no knowledge of depression or understanding of its clinical symptoms, I found myself deeply hurt, and running out of patience. Why was he inflicting such chaos on our lives? Why couldn't he sort himself out, snap out of it, come to his senses? Every cliché in the book . . . I thought it.

Things came to a head, as they are wont to do, with a trip home. Scott went back to Canada, to sort himself out. When he returned, ten days later, he was miraculously transformed.

I noticed the changes right away. At the airport, as the driver and I stood waiting by the arrivals gate, Scott spotted us in the crush of people and waved triumphantly. Gone was the furrowed brow and vacant stare. Gone were the hunched shoulders. Grinning broadly, he looked exhausted but otherwise content. More than content – he looked like he'd just felled a large tree or wrestled a wild beast, emerging unscathed. He looked supremely proud. Of himself.

I remember thinking, *I've never seen Scott look this way before.* Puzzled, I didn't know what to make of that observation.

Scott told me his doubts had been resolved, that for the first time in months he was truly happy. In Toronto, he said, he'd seen a psychologist who told him most people with his kinds of doubts require months, if not years, of therapy to work through them. But in rare cases, people can just snap out of it. Scott was convinced he was one of those rare few.

For me, Scott's drastic shift in mood came as a relief. But it was a relief tinged with doubt. The transformation seemed somehow too complete, too sudden. There was an intensity to Scott's new look, an urgency to his words, that seemed somehow too much.

The next day, at the bureau, Scott slung his arm around my shoulder and told the reporter and her husband that he'd turned a new leaf. He beamed with pleasure as he told them of his new-found happiness.

"That's great," they said. "Just great." I sensed they, too, were surprised. But no one said anything. We all just smiled.

If I was out of my element in understanding Scott's depression, I was *way* out of it regarding hypomania. I had no idea what I was dealing with. (Months later, in China, Scott's mother asked, by telephone, if I thought Scott might be manic-depressive. Incredibly, it was the first time I'd heard the term.)

For several weeks, I didn't say much about Scott's mood. It seemed odd to question happiness, to tell someone they have a little too much of it. So I tried to set my niggling doubts aside. The changes in Scott were benign enough that I could do so for days at a time. Scott has already described those changes: the need for less sleep; repeated assertions about his happiness; a tendency to talk too much, to dominate conversations.

And a desire to shop. That winter, Scott spent an increasing amount of time buying stuff. I'd never known him to be much of a shopper before. But now he bought kitchen appliances, a stereo system on a trip to London, Russian trinkets, rugs and artwork. None of it was exorbitantly expensive, and all of it was practical or pretty. But still. I noticed. I simply didn't know what to do or say about it.

When I did raise concerns – "We don't need that" – his sheer enthusiasm shot them down. "But we *want* it!" he'd exclaim. "We work hard, we live in a difficult city, why not indulge?"

It's hard to describe the magnitude of Scott's enthusiasms, the sheer force of his cheer. It was infectious, yes, but also overpowering. I felt like a party pooper, unable to have as much fun, see as much beauty or humour, as he did everywhere. Watching a decent video in our apartment, he'd declare it the best and funniest movie he'd ever seen. "That's hilarious, don't you think? Isn't it? It is!" Was I missing something? Was it really *that* funny?

Part of the problem was that we were so far from home, away from friends and family who might have noticed the changes, and reinforced my doubts. Nobody in Moscow knew Scott, knew he wasn't normally quite so joyous. They probably thought this was his true self, his personality freed from the grips of depression. That's certainly what he told everyone.

So, those first few months, I noticed changes, worried about them but was not overly consumed. I was working regularly by this point, and Scott was still spending most of his time at the bureau. So we had lots of time apart, and other things to focus on besides each other.

Over time, though, the changes grew more pronounced and became harder for me to rationalize. His drinking was especially troublesome. He drank only at night, after work, but always right up till bedtime. It was the source of many an argument.

"But if you're so incredibly happy, then why do you need to drink?"

Scott came up with lots of excuses – work was stressful, he was under pressure, he was trying to relax. None of them made sense to me, and I told him so, but to no avail. The more my concerns grew, the more defensive Scott became. By late spring, we were at an impasse: he could neither share nor comprehend my apprehensions, and I could neither share nor comprehend his relentless enthusiasms.

I remember discussing this with the correspondent who worked with Scott. She expressed concern that Scott seemed unapproachable, that he didn't want to listen to what anyone else had to say. I told her I'd been experiencing the same thing at home. We were both baffled, unsure what to do.

The confusing thing about mental disorder, to the uniniti-ated, is that it doesn't overtake the person entirely. Either someone is obviously disordered, you think, or they are obvi-ously not. Scott was neither.

Like the drinking, his fixation on sending messages late at night was contradictory. Again, I wondered, if he's so happy, why is he complaining so routinely to CBC management? He felt underappreciated, as if his talents, over the years, had not been recognized. This was somewhat understandable, but why now? Why such a surge of anger and resentment when life was supposedly so good?

A pattern set in. I would go to bed, because it was late, and I was tired, and I had to get up in the morning. Scott would stay up "just for a bit." When I'd wake up the next morning, tired and groggy, he'd already be up, wide awake. This in itself was mystifying. How could he not be tired? How could he need so little sleep? Then, he'd tell me sheepishly that he'd sent another message.

His message-sending was irrational; it defied logic or explanation. But when I pointed all this out to him, he would readily agree. "You're right. I shouldn't have sent the message. It was silly. And I'll stop. It won't happen again." At such moments, he was lucid and rational and reasonable. I couldn't make sense of the contrast.

I should state that at no time did it occur to me that Scott might have a diagnosable disorder. That did not seem remotely within the realm of possibilities. Here again, my ignorance was at work. He was working, he was happy, he was making sense most of the time. He wasn't delusional, talking to himself, hearing voices. He did not match my vague, uninformed picture of mental illness: if anything, I was the one who seemed ill.

In the couple of weeks before Scott's blow-up at the CBC, I found myself exhausted, nauseous, and weak. A trip to the doctor uncovered a number of problems: mononucleosis, an inflamed gall bladder, and pancreatitis. In retrospect, perhaps stress had taken a physical toll; at the time, I made no such connection. But I did take to my bed, slept a lot, and was placed on a strict diet.

Scott, meanwhile, was working incredibly long hours, preparing for the Yeltsin-Clinton summit. He would run in and out of the apartment, bringing food and medication for me, changing his clothes, talking a mile a minute. He seemed highly excitable, and full of ideas. His plan, I recall, was to work for one more year at the CBC, then quit his job and become an entrepreneur/inventor. Meanwhile, he was consumed with summit planning.

I can think of no worse combination than one person fuelled with hypomanic energy, and another slowed down by mononucleosis. It made for a strange household.

The most alarming moment for me, during all of this, was the evening Scott came home with that night-vision scope, purchased from a roadside kiosk. To me, he looked absolutely terrified. He came rushing into the apartment, wild-eyed and speaking urgently, convinced that someone had been following him. He asked me to lock the doors, look out the windows. Of course, there was no one there. Discovering that scope seemed crucially significant to him, but I could not remotely understand how or why.

This was the first time that I recall thinking something was seriously wrong. Scott was overwrought and could not be calmed. He looked strangely possessed; his whole body seemed overtaken. For the first time, I thought he needed to see a doctor.

But the next morning, the old pattern was back. I awoke to find Scott already up, and seemingly calm. He sat on the edge of our bed and told me I'd been right. In a reasonable voice, he explained that he'd overreacted, that he realized his discovery of the scope was no momentous coincidence.

I told him, again and again, that I was extremely concerned by what I'd witnessed. He could not explain why he'd been so upset, but in the end, I let him off the hook. I let myself be swayed. I let him convince me he was okay. I now see that as a crucial moment, a missed opportunity.

It's amazing what the human mind can rationalize. What had begun, several months earlier, as a desire to believe Scott was fine had turned into a desire to believe he would be fine, with time and rest. The alternative was just unfathomable.

In retrospect, a trip to China was probably the worst thing we could have done. A trip to the doctor, a full accounting of Scott's behaviour, was in order. At that time, he was probably still well enough to agree to it. Instead, I let Scott convince me that a change of environment, some time away from all of our troubles in Moscow, might help.

Scott and I have always loved to travel. A desire to see the world has been one of our strongest bonds. But travelling is stressful at the best of times, both physically and emotionally.

And there is no worse place to be, when someone you love is in crisis, than far from home, in a strange place, knowing no one.

In my memory, those weeks in China are one long marathon run through the streets of Beijing, trying to keep up with Scott. Which, of course, I couldn't. Never mind that I was in a city unlike any I'd ever seen, surrounded by a language I could not speak. Never mind that I was still recovering from my own illnesses. The truth is, it's impossible to keep up with someone who's manic. Their energy is boundless and unchecked.

In photographs from that trip, I look thin and exhausted. Scott was increasingly irritable, and we argued constantly. I couldn't win. Every argument I presented, every unacceptable behaviour I called him on, was quickly shot down. Scott, who is normally a calm and gentle soul, was upset with me for daring to disagree with anything he said. I could see the fury in his pinched face, in his penetrating eyes.

In Beijing, almost everything I knew and loved about Scott would vanish: his sharp wit, considerate nature, and eminent reasonableness. All this faded rapidly away. Instead, I found myself traipsing around Beijing with a loud-mouthed, sharp-tempered, pompous jerk. He was constantly in motion – talking, buying, making new friends. And downing vast quantities of alcohol.

People have told me they're amazed I didn't leave him. I admit that I was sorely tempted. Mania is one of the most exasperating states of mind you'll ever encounter. I can certainly understand why other spouses choose not to stay. Not knowing that his behaviour was the result of a disorder, I was sick to death of dealing with him. I'll just get back to Moscow with him, I told myself, and then we're through.

If we'd been anywhere but Beijing, I probably wouldn't have lasted as long as I did. I knew nothing about how the place worked, how to get anywhere, do anything on my own. Scott negotiated with taxi drivers and hotel owners, arranged plane tickets, dinners, and visits with his friends. He made quite a sight, racing around Beijing in his (newly purchased) baggy

Chinese pants, a thick necklace over his T-shirt, a Discman in one hand, headphone wires dangling from both ears. He played music constantly and loudly, no doubt to drown out my many complaints.

The Chinese were delighted and impressed by this outspoken Westerner, thrilled by his bold affection and grasp of the language. Scott was eager to talk with everyone. Small crowds would gather to listen to him speak.

"There must be lots of foreigners in Beijing who speak Mandarin. Why are they so astonished by Scott?" I asked a friend of his.

"Because he speaks Mandarin like us, like a Chinese person," she replied. Indeed, he spoke better Mandarin than when he lived in Beijing; his former colleagues told me so.

None of the Chinese we encountered – from old friends to strangers on the street – seemed to notice anything unusual about this different Scott. In fact, they all appeared quite taken with him. Perhaps they were merely being polite. I remember a flood of delighted smiles and applause when Scott took to the microphone during karaoke night at our hotel pub. He sang the first few lines of a local rock classic, in Mandarin, and then basked in the ensuing adulation. To Scott, I was the lone whiner, the sole disapproving stick-in-the-mud.

It was impossible to sleep at night while he prowled our hotel room, noisily awake. He was intent on videotaping our trip, and had purchased a projector that cast pictures onto walls. I remember waking up one morning to see a huge moving image of myself displayed on the ceiling above our bed.

"Isn't it great?" were the first words out of his mouth.

At a certain point, I let him wander the streets alone. I simply lacked the energy to keep up with him. Once, while Scott was out, a close friend of his called the hotel room. She was a kind and diplomatic Chinese journalist, and I told her how worried I'd become. She had noticed, she said, that Scott was not himself. "But what can you do? He will be better once he is home."

It had become impossible, by this point, to believe that. I knew something was seriously wrong; I just had no idea what it could be. Scott's parents were also alarmed, having been on the receiving end of many lengthy and excited late-night phone calls. I can only imagine what they felt, sitting in Saskatoon, listening to their son ramble from halfway around the planet. Eventually, I spoke to them myself, and we tried to figure out what was happening. This was when his mother mentioned manic depression, something a friend of hers had suggested.

This was new to me, the possibility of a diagnosis, an actual name for an actual disorder. Locking myself in the bathroom while Scott was in the bedroom playing with his camera gear, I called a friend in Canada. Her husband was a psychiatrist, the only one I knew. He asked me several specific questions: Was Scott's speech pressured? (Yes); How much was he sleeping? (A couple of hours a night); Was his manner grandiose? (Definitely so). After several more questions, he told me these were all the symptoms of mania.

"Will he be able to keep functioning?" I asked, confused. "Or is he headed for a breakdown?"

"He's already in one," was the stark reply.

My psychiatrist friend suggested that I not argue with Scott but gently try to convince him to see a doctor. "This will probably be your most difficult task," he said.

And of course, it was. Scott refused to believe there was anything wrong. It was inconceivable to him that he could be ill. I tried, as suggested, to emphasize how tired he was.

"It must be exhausting," I said, "having so little sleep."

Scott began to cry then, and conceded that he was, indeed, exhausted. He lay down on our hotel bed and held my hand to his chest, where his heart was furiously beating. He told me he feared cardiac arrest. I listened with a sudden surge of sympathy, and thought we might be making progress.

But in a moment, Scott was on his feet again, back on top of the world. No need for doctors. He came up with another solution. He would find some calming Chinese teas with herbs to "control the *Qi*."

One day, while Scott was out shopping, I called the CBC's Employee Assistance Plan in Toronto, and spoke with a social worker. The details of the conversation elude me, but it was clear that there was little they could do to help until we were back in Canada. I do remember her asking if Scott might become violent, if my safety could be at risk. "If so, get out of there," she said.

It was inconceivable to me that Scott could be violent. But the fact she'd even asked the question was terrifying. It made me painfully aware of how little I knew, how out of control the situation had become.

By this time, several of Scott's Canadian friends were involved, having also received phone calls from him. They, too, tried to convince him to see a doctor. One close friend, after a lengthy discussion, had Scott near to agreeing. But in the end, he refused.

Scott, meanwhile, was still joyously purchasing Chinese furniture. Initially, I'd thought this was not a bad idea. The tables, chairs, and beds we looked at were finely crafted, aesthetically pleasing, and unbelievably cheap. All I tried to do was limit the volume of his purchases. A few pieces would sell; many pieces might not.

But as Scott's mania built, my own influence shrank. Reasoning with him had become fruitless. And the furniture he was buying had, by then, become the least of my worries. Scott's rapid deterioration was a far more pressing matter. He was worsening by the day, losing more and more touch with reality.

In such dire circumstances, I tried to focus on what I could do. First, get him back to Hong Kong, where people at least spoke English, where I might somehow find help. Then, if possible, get back to Moscow two days later, on our scheduled flight.

The trip back to Hong Kong was inconceivably trying. Scott had bought so much stuff – clothes, trinkets, that damned projector – that our suitcases could not handle the load. We arrived at the airport with open sacks, overflowing with stray clothing. The ticket agent diplomatically provided masking tape. On the airplane, Scott talked and laughed to himself, rocked back and forth in his seat, and paced the aisle. He ordered several drinks. Passengers stared and the flight attendants looked worried.

I thought of how he'd been on the flight in: excited, chatty, and boisterous, but not unreasonable. The damage done in just two weeks, the sharpness of the descent, was overwhelming. It seemed impossible that he could survive the much longer trip from Hong Kong to Moscow without being punched out, arrested, or refused boarding.

In Hong Kong, things got worse. Scott decided he wanted to go to a Buddhist retreat and meditate. Coincidentally, there was a monastery on a nearby island that received visitors; Scott was determined to get there. The last ferry for the night, however, had already left. So he announced that he would stay there, by the river, until the next one arrived.

It took every ounce of my strength not to leave him there, walk back to a main street, hail a taxi, and check in to the nearest hotel. My presence seemed entirely unhelpful; he listened to nothing I said. He simply couldn't hear me. Scott's mind was overflowing, a veritable river of thoughts and emotions swollen past its banks. And in that noisy current, my own voice had grown distant, tiny, and irrelevant.

In the end, I couldn't bring myself to leave him. What might he do? Wherever would he wind up?

So I stayed. And somehow, improbably, we did make it to a hotel.

After a harrowing, sleepless night, I knew my options had been reduced to one. That morning, I told Scott what I was going to do. I left the room, rode the elevator to the main floor. At the front desk, I asked to speak to the manager. Did the hotel have a doctor on staff?

"No, but we can call one. Why? Are you ill?"

"No," I said. "But my husband is not well."

The woman gave me an inquiring look, and I tried not to cry. "He is acting strange," I said. "Not himself."

"Ah, yes," she said. "Was he in the lobby earlier? We saw a man here, dancing by himself. But we thought he must be drunk."

"He isn't well," I repeated. "I think he is very ill."

She promised to bring a doctor promptly.

Relieved, I returned to our room, imagining a kindly physician arriving with a stethoscope, perhaps a tranquillizer. A wise man who would appear in our doorway and fix this problem, make Scott well.

In fact, what the manager had called was an ambulance. When the paramedics showed up, I was shocked, but Scott looked not the least surprised. Somebody suggested I wait outside, as my presence seemed to distress him. In fact, he was assuring them the problem was all in my head.

I was out there, in the hallway, when I heard a loud thump.

"What's going on?" I said.

"Stay out here," the manager replied. "It is better for you."

The thump was, in fact, Scott punching a hole in a closet door. The door to the room opened and Scott described his feat for me proudly. Then the door closed again. Things quieted down; we could hear Scott talking. The hotel manager tried to make conversation: "He speaks Mandarin? Where did he learn that?" It was a surreal experience, out there in that hallway. I felt an intense pressure to behave normally, to speak reasonably, as if no horror was taking place.

When I finally went back inside, a paramedic was talking in a soothing voice while Scott lay tied to a stretcher. As they carried him out to the ambulance, Scott was miraculously calm, as if the voice had entranced him.

In the hospital examining room, two attendants stood by while we waited for the doctor. They laughed hilariously when Scott told them he was a "White Seeking Peace." I was outraged by their laughter – how could they be so insensitive, so cruel – but Scott seemed not remotely bothered.

When the doctor finally came, he was calm, confident, and efficient. After a brief conversation with Scott, and a few questions for me, he suggested transfer to a psychiatric hospital, for assessment and treatment. I would have to sign some papers – and the doctor would too – for Scott to be committed involuntarily. The doctor was certain this was the best plan.

I was so relieved that someone knew what to do – could help Scott in ways that I could not – that I readily agreed. We were standing by the nursing station, discussing the paperwork, when I noticed Scott wander out into the hallway in his purple hospital gown.

"Where's he going?" I asked, surprised.

The doctor looked over but seemed unconcerned. He returned his attention to the papers.

The next thing I knew, someone was shouting that Scott had left the hospital. I raced outside. Several hospital orderlies were also in hot pursuit, one of them with a wheelchair. But nobody seemed to know what to do. There was total confusion, chaos, lots of shouting. Just then, a train pulled up to the stop, the doors opened, and Scott ran on.

I don't remember how the police got there, but they seemed unwilling to get involved. They ordered the train stopped, kept the doors open, and just stood there, watching. A kind of standoff ensued. I was shouting, trying to get Scott off the train. Scott was shouting, saying he would sue anyone who made him go back to the hospital. He told them he was a journalist, a Canadian, and that his rights were being abused. The officers looked at each other nervously, and kept their distance.

Finally, I cornered one officer who spoke some English, and tried to explain that this man was not well, that he needed to be in the hospital.

"Has he been committed?"

"No, we were just in the process of doing that when he ran off."

"Then we cannot take him back there."

There was no doctor in sight, no one to confirm my story. Panic surged through me. I had visions of the train doors closing, of Scott vanishing into the centre of Hong Kong, barefoot, in his hospital gown, with no money or ID. I saw him jumping from a rooftop, or into the harbour, convinced he could fly or walk on water.

"Don't you understand?" I pleaded. "He can't leave here. He has to stay. He's very, very sick!"

It seemed Scott's life – his whole future – was in this officer's hands. The man paused, considering. It was true, he said, that Scott had no right to ride the train without a ticket. And he had no money to buy one. Finally, the order came: Take Scott off the train.

How to describe the pain I felt then? Scott was terrified, surrounded, completely alone. I, who should have been his ally, was making the officers do what terrified him most. But I could see no other option, no other safe way out.

"Take pictures!" Scott screamed at me, as they dragged him back to the hospital. "For evidence. Take pictures!"

I was running down the hospital hallway, into the room, when they injected Scott.

"What is that?" I asked.

"It is necessary," I was told. "It will calm him down. He will feel better."

Within minutes, Scott was asleep. For the first time in what seemed like days, he was actually still. I sat there, watching him breathe. At the foot of his bed, a clipboard bore his name and the words "severe psychosis." So that's what they call this, I thought. That's what has made him this way.

Later that day, the psychiatric hospital was another assault to the senses. This was a different world, completely unlike the clean and orderly general hospital. Patients clung to the huge fence surrounding the complex, looking heavily drugged, as if they hadn't seen the outside world in years. They called out to me, in a chorus of greetings, each time I entered the gate.

Inside, the rooms were dingy and decrepit. But the staff knew what they were doing. They talked to Scott at length, then to me. It would take time and observation to confirm a diagnosis, they said, but it was probably a mood disorder. I was so confused that my first thought was, Thank God. Only a mood disorder. Nothing serious. But they also mentioned schizophrenia; after all, there had been "auditory hallucinations." This was a whole new language – one I knew I must rapidly learn.

The doctor wanted information about Scott's medical history, and was particularly interested in his depression prior to Moscow and his use of an antidepressant. I told them what I could. I asked what I could think to ask. And then I was expected to leave.

Saying goodbye was, without doubt, the hardest thing I've ever done. Scott was sitting in the dreary nursing station, holding a mug of warm milk. What awaited him lay just beyond the observation windows: a row of hard beds, a dark room filled with patients.

How can I leave him here? I thought. How can I sleep in a hotel bed? I wanted to stay with him, to offer what comfort I might. Then Scott looked up. "It's nice here," he said quietly. "Don't you think?"

In that moment, I thought he was helping me, trying to ease my burden, my guilt. I'd been thinking he would hate me forever – had every right to – for what I'd done. Instead, he told me he would be okay here, with so many nice people.

The taxi ride back to the hotel – I could scarcely remember its name – was lonely in the extreme. For weeks, I'd been surrounded by noise, commotion, chaos, an overload of the senses. Now, suddenly, there was silence. Myself, alone, in silence, to think about what I'd done.

Our room had been quietly cleared out. I was expected to collect our things, pay the bill, and leave. No choice in the matter. I found a hotel closer to the hospital, and checked in.

The next few days were busy: notifying family, calling the CBC in London and Moscow, arranging for Scott's release. Phone calls to the hospital were frustrating, the updates on Scott's condition not nearly as informative as I wanted them to be. One morning, they said he'd been up most of the night, "disrupting some of the patients." There were no further details, and the staff had little time to answer my questions. But at some point, they confirmed the diagnosis: bipolar affective disorder. Whatever that meant.

When they told me Scott would be released, to spend a couple of days with me at the hotel before the flight home, I was terrified. How could I manage with him on my own? The drugs had slowed him down, but he was still manic, still not remotely like himself.

Lord knows how we must have looked as we stepped into the arrivals area of Saskatoon airport. I did not know Scott's family well, had just met his father. It was a strange kind of meeting, saying hello to these kind, concerned parents whose son I'd just had committed.

That night, a beautiful June evening, we had a family barbecue in the backyard. Scott's parents were there, his two sisters and one nephew. To an outsider, it would have looked for all the world like a happy family reunion. But there were many arrangements to be made; foremost among them, convincing Scott to go back into a hospital voluntarily. Scott's family had already arranged for the first step, a doctor's appointment.

Scott, however, was talking about going off his medication and returning to Toronto. Had that happened, he would have been committed: a traumatic undertaking for everyone and especially for Scott. But the hospital psychiatrist handled a delicate situation deftly. He held family meetings with Scott, and encouraged us to work together. He gave us information about bipolar disorder and its manic phase.

Scott was happy to answer the doctor's questions.

Doctor: "So you were in China?"

Scott: "Yes."

Doctor: "And you spent lots of money on Chinese furniture?"

Scott: "Yes."

Doctor: "And you have recently become a Buddhist?"

Scott: "Yup."

Doctor: "And you see nothing unusual about all this?"

We all leaned forward expectantly.

Scott (very confidently): "No."

I remember all of us – Scott's two sisters, his mother and father, his father's wife, and me – sitting on hard plastic chairs, clinging to the doctor's every word. We desperately wanted to be told what to do, how to make things better.

To me, it was an enormous relief to be with people who knew and cared about Scott, and who wanted to help. We were a kind of relay team, and I, exhausted from my race, was happily passing the baton.

And, in fact, that's pretty much what happened. Within a day or two I had succumbed to the Hong Kong flu, and while I lay in bed, drifting in and out of sleep, with a fever of 104°F, a minor miracle happened: Scott's father convinced him to enter the hospital voluntarily. Scott told me later that, although he did not believe he was ill, he acknowledged that if everyone in his family, individually, was encouraging him to enter hospital, there might be something to it.

In hospital, Scott was still flying high, seemingly unaffected by what staff told him. Sitting on a hospital patio one day, a nurse patiently explained how mood cycles worked, and what was considered a "normal" range of emotion. I lapped the information up, but Scott was barely listening. Another day, a social worker called and mentioned, in passing, the "special accommodations" that would have to be made for Scott's religion.

"What religion?" I asked.

"His Buddhism," she stated. "The fact he's been a Buddhist for seventeen years."

"He's been a Buddhist for about seven days," I told her.

The social worker fell silent briefly. "The smart ones," she said, "can be very convincing."

So there were moments of humour. But mostly there was panic, confusion, and extreme stress. Would Scott stay in hospital voluntarily? Would he keep taking his meds? When would he be his old self again? I missed Scott – the man I'd known and loved. It seemed I hadn't seen him in a very long time.

In times of crisis – when your world is falling apart – everyone needs a saviour. Someone who leaps into the fray and offers help without being asked. Someone whose presence makes you feel not quite so alone. And when your partner is in mental distress, you lose the very person who would normally fill that role. In Saskatoon, my saviour ended up being a woman I'd only just met: Kathy, who is married to Scott's dad. Kathy and I talked for hours on end, curled up on her couch, dissecting every detail of the day's developments (and there were always plenty). When I was sick, she provided cold compresses and fluids to break the fever. And when I was troubled, she spoke with wisdom, optimism, and good sense. Most of all, though, what she did was listen. Quietly, empathetically, and with respect. At a time when everyone's attention – including my own – was focused on caring for Scott, Kathy cared for me, too. And for that, I shall be forever grateful.

Even when misfortune was most extreme, then, we were lucky in lots of ways: a good doctor, a caring family, a supportive environment. I've learned that, sadly, this is not the norm.

While Scott was in hospital, I flew back to Moscow, packed our bags, and emptied our apartment. A thankless task filled with sad memories and an overwhelming sense of loss. Too much had happened; I could not assimilate it all. And the future seemed so uncertain.

People keep telling me that I'm so brave, so strong, that I'm handling it all so well, I wrote in my journal. *But most of all, what I am is numb. . . . I want someone else to take care of things for me but there is no one. Is this the equivalent of shell shock?*

By the time I returned to Canada, two weeks later, Scott's mania had subsided. I'd learned that a depression often followed a manic episode, but as we prepared to return to Toronto, I was sure the worst was over.

If mania is infuriating to deal with, severe clinical depression is truly heartbreaking. It's like watching someone you love being held down and beaten raw, one punch at a time. The pain is that intense, the torment that relentless. And you are powerless to help, a ghostly witness to so much suffering.

My most enduring image is of Scott, lying in bed with a pillow propped over his forehead, eyes, and nose. Every time I climbed the stairs, I did so with dread, knowing I would find him there, wide awake and infinitely troubled, blocking out the light, the outside world. When I peeled off the pillow, I knew exactly what I'd see: pain, in those two blue eyes, in that sad, sad face. The gloom just poured off him, surrounding him like some hideous, dark aura. It filled our apartment, and threatened to overtake me too.

I'd read many books by now, and knew more about the disorder. But I still knew nothing about the services. Where to get help? Who to ask? We'd left Saskatoon with no follow-up plan for his hospital stay. And he had no family in Toronto, only me.

In *my* family, there was some unexpected news. Scott and I had scarcely returned from Saskatoon when the phone rang: my father had had a major heart attack. Over the next few months, while Scott was depressed in Toronto, my father was on a waiting list for bypass surgery in Ottawa. As daughter *and* spouse, my stress levels went through the roof. And yet I chose not to share this with my family. They were already worried about my father; I was loathe to have them worry about me, too. I also felt enormously protective towards Scott, because none of my family knew him well. They hadn't seen much of the charming, witty soul I had once fallen for. If I divulged the grimmest details of his depressed self, would they understand that this was not the *real* Scott? The longer his depression dragged on, the more reticent I became. I'm sure

my family did not understand the enormity of Scott's suffering, or mine, until his story appeared in the *Toronto Star*.

I focused on finding some professional help for Scott. His
GP had recommended some psychiatrists, but Scott was simply
incapable of making phone calls, arranging appointments.
And finding doctors for someone else, I discovered, was tricky.
There were long waiting lists, and lots of roadblocks. "Why
are *you* placing the call?" "He'll have to book something
himself."

In the end, I phoned the psychologist Scott had seen
months before, on his return trip to Toronto from Moscow.
I was surprised when he phoned me back and let me tell him
about Scott's condition. He even suggested we both attend the
first session.

That session ended up helping me more than Scott. The psychologist practised cognitive-behavioural therapy, which focuses
on breaking down negative thought patterns. He outlined his
approach: over many months, Scott would come to terms with
his illness, allow himself to move on. He compared bipolar
disorder to a physical illness, from which recovery was fully
possible. It seemed like an eminently reasonable plan.

But Scott felt the psychologist was trivializing his experiences, not acknowledging the trauma he'd suffered. He did not
return. And I learned an important lesson: I could not will
Scott into treatment, nor make choices for him.

So, after weeks of searching, we were back to square one.
No doctor in sight. One night, I dragged Scott out to see a
movie with a friend who was visiting from Ottawa. It took
a massive amount of energy for Scott to step out the door, let
alone chat with friends. But I encouraged him to try. I'd noticed
that, sometimes, when Scott forced himself outside, his mood
did improve slightly. But not this time. Scott sat in black silence
while the audience laughed uproariously; the movie was a
comedy. And right afterwards, he told me he had to go home.
His face was wretched; I knew he would go straight to bed.
But he encouraged me to stay, to go on to the pub where we'd
arranged to meet more friends.

There, I sat with three of Scott's best buddies. They asked how he was, why he hadn't come. They knew, of course, about the depression. But they didn't know how bad – how all-consuming – it had become. I was the only person besides Scott who really knew, who saw the toll it took day after day.

I've never been good at asking for help. But that night, I did. I asked, tearily, if we could pool our resources to find a good doctor. And within a few days, one of them had come up with a name, someone who specialized in bipolar disorder and was actually taking on new patients.

If this seemed like the solution to all our problems, it wasn't. There were no quick fixes. In fact, Scott got worse before he got better. But at least a specialist could monitor Scott's mood, try different combinations of drugs, give him the best that medicine had to offer. At least he had someone qualified to talk to, someone he trusted, who had far more expertise than me. When Scott started having suicidal thoughts, he told her as well as me. And this was hugely reassuring, knowing that she could step in when needed.

Scott's "suicidal ideation," as I came to know it, was terrifying for me. Every time I stepped out of the house, I worried that he might act on his visions of death. Scott kept promising he wouldn't, but I knew how thankless a task life had become.

After discussing it with Scott, I called his doctor, and told her of my fears. She recommended a hospital stay. Scott was reluctant to go; I was uncertain how it might help. We were both crying as a nurse led him onto the psych ward, less than six months after he'd last left one. In fact, we were lucky to have found a bed, so limited were the spaces. But this was December, and several patients were leaving for Christmas holidays.

The hospital stay did seem to help, if only by providing a brief escape from the pressures of the outside world. I got some help for myself, too. Through the CBC's Employee Assistance Plan, I visited a therapist, who told me I was at risk of becoming depressed myself. Aside from trying to help Scott, I was readjusting to life in Canada, looking for work, managing the Chinese furniture business. Emphasizing the importance of maintaining my own health, she told me depression could be contagious. She encouraged me to take daily walks alone, visit friends, do something each day that gave me pleasure. Most of all, she filled the kind of role that Kathy had in Saskatoon: someone who saw me as my own person, with my own life to care for.

With time, over many months, I developed a profound respect for Scott. For his ability to endure. I knew how hard it was just waking up each day. I knew how deeply this diagnosis had dug into his sense of self. Each time he entered hospital, swallowed a pill, or told one more person his story, I knew how deeply he was drawing on reserves. But still he kept going. In his shoes, I'm not sure I could have walked so far.

Depression and mania share one thing in common: a certain self-absorption that can look selfish and ungrateful. As the caring partner, it seems your own role – the support you provide, the pain you feel – amounts to nothing. You give and give, and you don't get a lot in return.

Each night, Scott thanked me, tearfully, for standing by him. He knew how draining this was for me, and his thanks was all he had to offer.

Telling yourself that this is caused by the disorder, not by anyone's failings, can help – but it doesn't resolve the central imbalance. The payoff comes later, when recovery is complete.

And I clung to that faith, that Scott would one day be well. From my reading, I knew that mood disorders are highly treatable. More importantly, though, I knew Scott. Unwell as he was, his true self still existed. The qualities that had brought him so much success in life – tenacity, talent, confidence – were all still in him. They had kept him alive through his despair, and they would help him become well.

The hard part was in getting there, in waiting and hoping, and seeing no progress. Days and weeks and months with this third party in our home – this dark and stubborn force that would not release its hold. Patience has never been my strong suit, but I learned its virtues in that time with Scott.

When times were at their worst, a couple of well-intentioned friends suggested I leave him. (No doubt, others thought the same but chose not to say so.) They were only thinking of my future, my best interests. But I can safely say now that those interests were best served by staying put. I have no regrets about choosing to take that journey, beside Scott. Disorder or not, there is no one quite like him. And I know that if the roles are ever reversed, he will do the same for me.

We live ordinary lives now, with jobs, a house, two cats, and weekends at the cabin. But we live, too, with the possibility of relapse, something I have troubled over more than Scott has. In the past, I leapt at each minor shift in mood, expecting the worst. Quite frankly, it was exhausting living that way. And so, after much discussion, I have accepted Scott's decision to be medication-free. He has accepted the need to manage his life with care. And with these agreements, with time, I have allowed myself to stop living in fear. Together, we plan for the future, and assume the best is yet to come.

HEATHER'S STORY

My dad was diagnosed with bipolar disorder about six years ago, when I was in my late teens. At the time, I was living at home with my mom, dad, and younger sister. Prior to the diagnosis, I was not aware that my dad had a mental health problem. But my mother and I knew something was definitely wrong. We knew that people do not usually experience the drastic fluctuation in moods that my father did.

When he was suffering from a depressive episode, he slept more, rarely got out of bed, and spoke from a narrow and depressed frame of mind. During his manic episodes, he would increase his spending, need very little sleep, and speak rapidly with racing thoughts and ideas. His depression/mania followed a seasonal pattern. He would begin to get depressed in early fall, and show signs of mania during spring. I hated the depression, and the mania scared me.

My father was often in denial that he had a problem, and thought the problem was with everyone else. When he was ill, it was difficult for him to recognize the symptoms of the disorder. He was finally diagnosed because the symptoms became harder for him to control. They got progressively worse with age, and the changes in his behaviour became more apparent. At the advice of a co-worker, my mother suggested that my father see a doctor. Both my mother and father went together, and my father was finally diagnosed.

I was relieved that the problem was finally identified, but it also brought mixed emotions and the thought that "my father has a mental illness." I was worried other people would find out and judge my father and me. I did not understand what the label meant, or what the prognosis was. I did not understand what it felt like for my father, if this was a permanent, untreatable disorder, or if this changed the person and father he was before the diagnosis.

Even with the diagnosis, my father initially had difficulty accepting that he had a mental disorder. When he was feeling well, he would stop taking his medication, believing that he did not need it.

I got a degree in psychology, believing that I could help my father. With education came an understanding and compassion towards my father and his illness. But at the same time, it created an obsession – his problems became my problems. When he was depressed, I went crashing down with him. I worried that he would take his own life and about how that would devastate our family. When he was manic, I worried about his safety due to his reckless behaviour. When my dad was very sick, I had difficulty focusing my energy on anything but him.

A turning point occurred for me last year. I got a call that my dad was experiencing a very difficult depressive episode and was not taking care of himself. When I first heard the news, I became very upset, but then I got angry. I was angry because it seemed like the same thing happened every year. My father would be doing great, and then he'd go off his medication and become very sick. I would wonder with each episode whether he would make it through. I was angry at him, and I was angry at the illness. I made up my mind that I would not let this pattern repeat itself for me.

I wrote my dad a letter and told him how his illness affected me. I told him I finally realized that I was not the one to take care of him. From now on, all I can do is offer my love, support, *and provide him with information. It is up to him what he does with that information, but at least I know in my heart that I did all I could. I was playing two roles – caregiver and daughter – and I choose to be his daughter.*

My father appreciated my honesty. He had not realized how much his illness had affected me. We now communicate more openly, and this incident has strengthened our relationship.

This story concludes with a happy ending, in large part because of the support and knowledge I received from the staff and volunteers at the Mood Disorders Association of Toronto and Ontario. Their motto is "Helping others help themselves." With their help, I was able to help my dad. I was able to talk openly with other family members and learn from their experiences, and they helped support my own decisions as well. The education I received there helped me dispel the stereotypes and myths associated with mental illness, and the fear of having a loved one diagnosed.

Today, I have a positive outlook for my father as well as my family. There are some painful memories that I would like to forget, but at the same time I can use them as a measure of success, because my dad is doing so much better now. He has a lot of courage and strength, and this has helped him to accept his illness. Now that he is doing well, I can have a loving relationship with the father that I always knew was there.

CHAPTER THREE

Your Story – It's More Common Than You Think

Name: Jean
Age: 27
Diagnosis: Depression

Jean had a rocketing career in the investment business in Western Canada. A good income, a wide circle of friends, and a man she still describes as "the love of my life."

Several years back, the love of her life killed himself.

Jean coped. She got past the shock, the funeral. She kept working and took up running, pounding the pavement obsessively for miles a day. And then, a year after his death, it started to fall apart.

"My parents thought I was being lazy because I was lying around on the couch," she says. "I was actually thinking of dying."

Her depression darkened. She left her job. She remained in bed most of the day, for months on end. An attractive woman who had previously paid a great deal of attention to clothes, she now wore a bland uniform of sweatpants and a sweatshirt.

Her physical health, over time, came to mirror her state of mind. She was perpetually exhausted.

"I just couldn't move," she says. "And when I *did* feel well enough to do things, I started to clean up my affairs so that if I killed myself, things would be easier."

She attended a hospital day-treatment program in an effort to climb out of the pit. She worked hard with a therapist, realizing there were issues in her own life beyond the grief that needed resolving. She refused all attempts to improve her condition with antidepressants.

"I want to get out of this on my own," she insists. "If I can make it through this, I believe I'll be a better person, a stronger person.

"If I can make it through this," she emphasizes, "I'll make it through anything."

Occasionally, bits of the old Jean flash through. The easy laugh, the sharp wit, the dancing eyes.

Those moments are elusive. They're more frequent now than they were. But they do not come often enough.

Though the name is a pseudonym, Jean is real. And while she may feel like she's alone, she's not. Depression causes more disability worldwide than any other single cause. A startling number of Canadians have experienced that same dark anguish; a 1994 study conducted for the Canadian Mental Health Association concluded that three million Canadians had symptoms of depression.

Which is why this chapter is *your* story, a snapshot of the astonishing impact of mental disorder in Canada and around the world. There will be some surprising statistics over the next few pages. But behind each statistic are faces. Of people like Jean. Maybe even you, or someone you love.

Getting a handle on the impact of mental disorder is never an easy task. A number of factors complicate the gathering of reliable data, not the least of which is stigma. Many people fear admitting to others, even to themselves, that their mental health may be suffering. The vast majority do not seek help of any kind, even though it can often immeasurably improve their lives. Some wrongly blame themselves for their mental discomfort; many may well be unaware anything is even wrong.

The information that follows will dispel some of the myths and replace them with facts. And the blunt fact is, mental disorder is so common that it will almost certainly strike someone close, perhaps very close, to you.

THE GLOBAL BURDEN

Ever wonder how many people have their lives cut short or are disabled by the world's big problems? War, disease, famine? The people at the World Health Organization (WHO) have wondered, too. And they, along with Harvard and the World Bank, tried to find some answers.

In a monumental study, the group attempted to measure what it called "The Global Burden of Disease." An unenviable task – especially since the trio wanted to create a new standard for meaningfully determining that burden. It would attempt, on a worldwide basis, to gauge how much disability leading "diseases" caused.

It decided, in the end, on two measures: DALYs and YLDs. The former stands for Disability Adjusted Life Years. It means, essentially, one lost year of healthy life, either through disability or premature death. It's a useful measure, in that it *totals* the years of healthy living lost to various diseases or disasters. (A young person killed or injured in a car crash would have a higher DALY score than would an elderly person, who had fewer productive years of life remaining.)

Although it was developed primarily as a tool for policy planners, the DALY chart is instructive. The sheer magnitude of the raw numbers may be too great to grasp, but what's useful is their ranking. Five of the top ten causes of DALYs, worldwide, are psychiatric disorders.

Leading DALY Causes, Ages 15–44, Worldwide (1990)

		Total (thousands)	Per cent of total
1)	Unipolar major depression	42,972	10.3
2)	Tuberculosis	19,673	4.7
3)	Road traffic accidents	19,625	4.7
4)	Alcohol use	14,848	3.5
5)	Self-inflicted injuries	14,645	3.5
6)	Bipolar affective disorder	13,189	3.1
7)	War	13,134	3.1
8)	Violence	12,955	3.1
9)	Schizophrenia	12,542	3.0
10)	Iron-deficiency anemia	12,511	3.0

From Christopher J.L. Murray and Alan D. Lopez, *The Global Burden of Disease* (1996) (table 5.4, page 270). Reproduced by permission.

More than 40 *million* years of life lost to death or disability by depression alone. And that's in just one age group, in one diagnostic category. By this measurement, depression exacts a toll on human life three times greater than war. It's hard to fathom.

And hard to ignore. Because the other big measure – the Years Lived with Disability (YLD) – tells a similar story: depression is once again at the top of the list for the same age group. An excerpt from the report published by the group warns that "the burden of psychiatric conditions have been heavily underestimated [in the past]. . . . Depression alone was responsible for more than one in every ten years of life lived with a disability worldwide."

It's worth noting that both schizophrenia and bipolar affective disorder – which affect far fewer people than does depression – also make the top ten. That's because both these disorders can involve prolonged and intense suffering for those afflicted.

Schizophrenia directly affects at least 221,000 people (1996 estimate) in Canada; recent estimates by the Schizophrenia Society of Canada place the figure at 300,000. People with this disorder occupy 8% of all hospital beds in Canada at any given time, and they tend to stay longer in hospital even than those with the most serious physical ailments.

Bipolar affective disorder affects a similar number of people. And while it tends to be more manageable than schizophrenia, episodes of mania and depression can be terribly destructive. Recent research indicates that these disorders affect more people than once thought. It's been estimated that as many as one million Canadians have what is often contentiously termed a "serious mental illness."

We'll dive into the debate over language, over the nature of mental disorders, later in the book. For the moment, however, let's agree that people suffer, for whatever reason, from issues of mental health that impair their lives.

A lot of people.

A TALE OF THREE STUDIES

Only a handful of attempts have been made to measure what could truly be described as the national mood. But what they've found is remarkably consistent: we're not in great shape.

The Ontario Mental Health Supplement, the largest single survey devoted exclusively to the topic in this country, took the mental pulse of nearly ten thousand people aged fifteen and older. It attempted to determine, based on a questionnaire administered in 1990–91, what kinds of disorders were present in the sample and how common (or uncommon) they were.

You may well wonder how a questionnaire could possibly tell us if a person has a disorder. The short answer is that it does so by asking the same kinds of questions a doctor would ask you.

In the Ontario Supplement, most of the questions were based on something called the Composite International Diagnostic Interview, or CIDI. This is a tool developed by the World Health Organization and used in measuring the frequency of mental disorders in the general population. When the answers to a series of yes-or-no questions are crunched by a software program, the results have been shown to agree closely with the diagnosis a clinician would make in person.

Among the study's findings:

- 19% of Ontarians aged fifteen to sixty-four years met the criteria for one or more mental disorders during the previous year;
- in the late adolescent/young adult age group, *one in four* had at least one disorder during the previous year;
- 75% of Ontarians with a mental disorder in the previous year did not seek help of any kind.

Although the work was limited to Ontario, the problem is not. One of the work's principal investigators, research scientist Dr. Paula Goering, says you'd find similar results pretty much anywhere in the country.

"The basic overall prevalence rates of around 20% of the population having some kind of disorder in any one year," says Dr. Goering, "are pretty consistent from study to study."

Which brings us to study Number Two, a comprehensive survey conducted in Western Canada. Dr. Roger Bland, Chair of the Department of Psychiatry at the University of Alberta, analyzed the data from interviews conducted with 3,258 people in Edmonton. The result?

"Our one-year prevalence," he says, "was 21%."

There's more. When the Alberta respondents were asked if they'd *ever* experienced symptoms of mental disorder in their lifetime (what's known as "lifetime prevalence"), the number jumped to 33.8%, a finding also consistent with other major studies. Meaning one in three of us is likely to experience what could be termed a mental disorder of some kind, at some point in our lives.

"Mental disorders," says Dr. Bland, "are probably commoner than people anticipate."

Read enough of these studies and you'll see another clear trend emerge: rates of disorder differ by gender. Men are far more prone to alcohol abuse than women, while women report symptoms of depression and anxiety far more frequently than men. There's another important difference: women, in virtually every study, are more likely to seek professional support. Men tend to suffer in silence, no doubt a contributing factor to their higher rates of suicide and alcohol abuse.

While the Alberta and Ontario studies offer a wealth of data, they don't tell us a whole lot about what happens over extended periods of time. We get a momentary glimpse – a freeze-frame – but we don't know what happens to these people after the interviewer folds up the questionnaire and leaves.

That's where longitudinal studies come in. These are designed to follow populations, and individuals within those populations, over longer time frames. They can tell us, for example, how many people recover and how many do not. They can track changing socio-economic variables, looking for their relationship with mental disorder. And the longest-term work of this kind, anywhere in the world, has been taking place in Canada.

The Stirling County Study was designed in 1948 by psychiatrist Dr. Alexander Leighton, a man with a particular interest in the relationship between the socio-cultural environment and mental health. He chose an area of Atlantic Canada and, for confidentiality reasons, gave it the fictitious name of Stirling County. The people in this region, of course, are very real. And researchers have been tracking their progress since 1952. At the moment, the study involves more than four thousand residents, some of whom have been monitored since the very outset. It, too, has found a consistent prevalence rate of 20%.

The current director of the project is its founder's wife, research scientist Dr. Jane Murphy of Harvard. And of all the data the Stirling County Study has generated, one finding, she believes, is perhaps the most significant.

"I think our most important finding concerns the outcome for depression," she says. "We ourselves, as investigators – and I think few others – had any idea how serious a disorder it is.

"About 78% of the people who were depressed in our first study [1952] had a poor outcome by 1968. By poor outcome, I mean they remained chronically or recurrently ill, either with a depression or they crossed over to anxiety. Men tended to remain depressed, and the death rates among men were significant. Twice as many depressed men died as one would expect relative to the entire male population."

Although that may sound bleak, it's important to note that the Stirling County Study was not designed to evaluate people who sought and followed treatment and compare them with those who did not, nor to measure which treatments were most beneficial. That kind of work requires a clinical trial, comparing under strict conditions a treated group of people against an untreated group with the same disorder. (Such trials do, incidentally, show more optimistic outcomes for those in appropriate treatment. There's also little doubt that treatment options have advanced dramatically in recent years.)

The data from Atlantic Canada shows consistent prevalence rates over time for each of the most common disorders. Depression affects about 5% of the adult population, anxiety another 5%. The first study indicated about 5% of the population was abusing alcohol, and other disorders – schizophrenia, bipolar affective disorder, Alzheimer's, etc. – account for the remaining 5%.

So, we've got three huge studies of Canadian populations, in three different regions, with the same result. One in five adult Canadians, in any given year, will meet the psychiatric criteria for a mental disorder. (The abuse of alcohol and other substances can meet the criteria for mental disorder.)

What's interesting is that many people in all three studies met the criteria for one *or more* mental disorders. Folks with anxiety were often drinking too much, or suffering from depression, or even all three.

When an additional disorder enters the equation, be it mental or physical, it's often referred to as a "dual diagnosis" or "co-morbidity." The most common dual diagnosis is the coexistence of a mental disorder along with alcohol abuse or dependence. Dr. Nady el-Guebaly, past president of the Canadian Psychiatric Association, specializes in this at his Calgary practice.

"The wisdom at the moment," he says, "is that about one-third of the population of people who are alcoholics and one-third of the general mental disorder population share a co-morbidity," he says. "And that proportion increases to about 50% for those who are using drugs other than alcohol."

When speaking of "disorder," the concept of impairment is key. All of us have troubles, issues, conflicts that roam our heads, but usually those thoughts are not invasive enough to start messing with other aspects of our lives. We deal with them and move on; we cope. When these thoughts or behaviours start to significantly impair our lives, they qualify as disorder.

WHO'S AT RISK?

Although the Ontario Mental Health Supplement was not designed to determine what *caused* mental disorders, its data did point out that certain associated circumstances – known as "risk factors" – appear to play a significant role.

Risk factors give us a useful clue as to who may be at risk of developing a disorder, but they don't predict who will. A useful analogy is to think of smoking as a risk factor for lung cancer. Those who smoke are at far greater risk of developing the disease – although some heavy smokers will continue puffing into their nineties without a problem. The same concept applies to mental health.

On the flip side of the coin, the *absence* of a risk factor is no guarantee things will be fine. Sometimes lung cancer strikes the person you'd least expect – the fitness buff with no family history of the disease. In the same fashion, so too can schizophrenia strike someone when there were no overt indicators they may be at risk.

Risk factors, then, can be thought of as weak links in a mental health chain. Sometimes those links will hold just fine; sometimes they won't.

One of the most consistent risk factors in the scientific literature is family history. Sixty-one per cent of people reporting symptoms of two or more co-existing disorders said they had a parent with a mental disorder. This is not to suggest that mental disorders are necessarily passed along in the same predictable manner as blue eyes or blonde hair, but parents can certainly be part of that chain.

The risk that a link may give also increases if a person was abused as a child. In the Ontario Supplement, 38% of those reporting two or more mental disorders also reported experiencing severe childhood abuse. "A strong potential determinant of mental disorder," reads the Supplement, "is the experience of serious physical and/or sexual abuse as a child. The exact way in which being mistreated as a child leads to mental disorders in adulthood is not known, and the investigation of this issue should receive high priority."

Of course, not every person who develops a mental disorder was traumatized as an infant or grew up in a dysfunctional family. That is clearly not the case. But this example of a risk factor does help emphasize a sometimes-neglected fundamental: many people become unwell because of very real things that happened in their lives.

Two other frequently cited risk factors for mental disorders are having a low income or living on public assistance. At the moment, however, there is no scientific consensus on the predominant *sequence* of events in these cases. In other words, did the person develop a disorder, lose their job, and then wind up on public assistance? Or did they lose

their job for some reason, have to sell their home, then become depressed?

We've met many people who would fit either category. And,
over a period now spanning nearly fifty years, the Stirling
County Study has found pretty much the same thing.

"We looked at incidence among people in the lower,
average, and the high socio-economic levels," says Dr.
Murphy. "And incidence was definitely higher among poorer
people. We interpreted that to suggest that there's something
about the environment, among adults at least, that's leading
to the emergence of a new disorder.

"But we also then took everybody who was depressed at
the beginning and looked to see where they ended up in terms
of the socio-economic scale. And there was a definite trend for
people with chronic, serious depression to drift downward in
the socio-economic hierarchy. So our interpretation, given the
limitations of our data, suggests that it's some of both."

What is crystal clear is that the people who are the health-
iest in Canada – mentally and physically – are those who have
the most in life. The highest incomes, the best educational
opportunities, the best nutrition. A major 1999 report on
Canada's population, *Toward a Healthy Future*, notes the dis-
parity in its opening pages. "Low-income Canadians are more
likely to die earlier and to suffer more illnesses than Canadians
with higher incomes, regardless of age, sex, race and place of
residence," it states. "At each rung up the income ladder,
Canadians have less sickness, longer life expectancies and
improved health."

And that includes mental health. Using data from the
1996–97 National Population Health Survey, the report found
the following: "For both men and women, the risk of depression was highest among those with the lowest incomes.
Thirteen per cent of women in the lowest income group were
at risk of depression, compared with 5% of women in the
highest income group. For men, the rate of depression ranged
from 11% among those in the lowest income bracket to 4%
among men with high incomes."

The report also notes disturbing rates of suicide, depression, and behavioural problems among Canada's young people. And while some of these problems show a link with household income level, others do not.

"Young women aged 15 to 19 years were the most likely of any sex-age group to exhibit signs of depression. Young Canadians aged 18 and 19 were the most likely to report high life stress levels (37%), compared to the national rate of 26%."

There will be much more on the nature/nurture debate in the following chapter. But our collective experience, including more than two hundred interviews with consumers, survivors, and mental health professionals, has taught us a simple truth: mental disorders are as individual as the people who live with them. There is no one single, simple cause.

For the purposes of this section, the debate is irrelevant. Because whether it was nature or nurture – or a head-on collision of both – the circumstances were beyond the control of the individual. No one *chooses* to have a mental disorder.

SEEKING HELP

The Ontario Supplement reported that more than a million people in that one province were afflicted with a mental disorder. Yet only one in four of them sought help of any kind – a ratio similar to that found in Alberta. Stigma, at least according to the Ontario study, played a clear role. Of those who had untreated disorders, more than half said they were too "embarrassed" to seek help.

Our dismal record in seeking help contrasts sharply with the high priority we say we place on our mental well-being. A 1997 Canadian Mental Health Association study carried out by the COMPAS research firm found that 82% of those surveyed felt their mental health was "very" important. That number was one of the highest "intense opinion" scores ever recorded by COMPAS in any of its attitudinal or behavioural studies.

So we care about our mental health. A mental disorder will eventually affect one in three of us. Yet only a minority reach out.

Slowly, that picture is changing. Canadians are increasingly choosing to seek help. And our decision to do so often seems to be sparked when the media tackles mental health issues in a responsible way. Whenever informative articles hit the press, the phone lines at the Mood Disorders Association of Canada (MDA) headquarters in Winnipeg, for example, become jammed.

"Every time the topic is mentioned in public, our phones light up," says MDA president Bill Ashdown. "And it tells us, again and again and again, that there is a huge underlying population of people who are in real need."

A population that includes health-care professionals.

"I couldn't tell you the number of doctors that we've sneaked in the back door," says Ashdown, "who come to see me at the house on weekends, who phone me at three in the morning – simply because they need help, but they can't afford to be recognized. It's a devastating comment on the openness, or lack of openness, in certain aspects of the medical profession."

In fact, the president of the Canadian Psychiatric Association is well aware of the problem. Dr. Michael Myers sees it every day in British Columbia, where he specializes in treating physicians with mental disorders.

"We've come some ways in overcoming stigma in the general public in North America," he observes, "but we've still got a ways to go in the medical field."

There are clear ways to determine if you need help, and where to go if you do. The many options will be covered in later chapters.

THE COSTS

In some ways, it's impossible to assess the personal cost of a mental disorder. How do you calculate the price of suffering?

What dollar figure eases the cruelty and discrimination of stigma? How much money would a person pay to be freed from suicidal thoughts? What value do we place on promise unfulfilled?

Those questions, of course, can never be truly answered. But in terms of the things we *can* measure, the cost is staggering. It adds up to billions and billions of dollars in Canada – the cost of direct health care, lost income, social support programs, medications, and more. According to the Canadian Institute for Health Information, people with mental disorders spent a total of more than five and a half *million* days in this country's hospitals in 1995–96. That's more than twice the number of days spent in hospital by people with all forms of cancer. In 1996, it was estimated that suicide resulted in 110,210 years of potential life lost – fourth in a list topped by cancer, accidents, and heart disease.

Even when you look at a single diagnosis, schizophrenia, the costs are formidable. A major paper by some of the country's most respected researchers pegged the direct health care costs (and non-health-care costs, such as group homes) at $1.12 billion in 1996. Another $1.23 billion in lost productivity (including premature death) was calculated, for a total of $2.35 billion that year. Factor in the burden placed on families, often the primary caregivers, and the figure climbs even higher. Some estimates of the annual economic cost of schizophrenia in Canada have approached $5 billion.

So immense is the impact that a group called the Canadian Business and Economic Roundtable on Mental Health is trying to make mental health a priority on the corporate agenda. Its president, Bill Wilkerson, has researched the topic extensively and is co-author, along with Dr. Edgardo Pérez, of *Mindsets – Mental Health: The Ultimate Productivity Weapon*. (See Appendix.)

Wilkerson says businesses that ignore mental health do so at their peril. "The economic impact of depression in the North American Free Trade Zone minus Mexico," he says, "is equivalent to an annual cost to business in excess of 50 billion dollars."

That figure includes lost productivity by people who are on the job but may be suffering from forms of anxiety that we often underestimate as "workplace stress." Frequently, says Wilkerson, that anxiety is induced by the workplace *itself*, particularly in environments where people feel they're little more than insignificant cogs in vast uncaring machines. In such surroundings, both the employees and their employers are losing out.

"You're talking about people," says Wilkerson, "who are reaching a stage where anxiety is compromising their ability to concentrate, compromising their ability to relate to other people well, and compromising their capacity to deliver consistently in the workplace."

And it's not just anxiety. A huge survey carried out by Westinghouse Electric Corporation in the late 1980s found that about 9% of male workers and 17% of female workers had experienced a major depressive episode in the previous year. The employees linked those depressions with specific workplace triggers, including "conflicting work demands, unclear job expectations and responsibilities, lack of intrinsic rewards, and negative job events."

But that's just part of the picture. Wilkerson, who also knows the health-insurance business intimately, says anywhere from one-third to one-half of all people who are off work and collecting disability are doing so for reasons of mental health. And he says even people who are off for *physical* reasons can find their recovery impeded by mental ill-health.

"When people are home, often on short-term disability with a low back injury or a soft tissue injury, there's a terrific emotional component to that thing," he says. "That is a painful, lonely, mentally wearing experience – and it is the source of a terrific amount of emotional distress. And people who go through that alone are people who take longer to get well."

WELLNESS

Amidst all these statistics it is easy to lose sight of the fact that people *do* get well. Indeed, given the chance, many thrive. Some of the brightest, most talented, most enthusiastic people we have met have been labelled "crazy." Not just crazy, but useless. Stupid.

Journalist and advocate Nora McCabe recalls how she felt the moment her son was diagnosed with schizophrenia. "It's almost as if they tell you that not only does he have this mental illness," she says bitterly, "but he's become a total moron. There's no expectation of function, or reintegration so that you can have any sort of a life a middle-class person would identify as successful or fulfilling."

McCabe and others with insight look beyond the disorder and see something wonderful. They see that the person never truly went away. They see a son with a desire to work, a brother with a sense of humour, a friend who still enjoys a coffee.

The most innovative – arguably some of the most successful – mental health strategies are those that recognize this. Programs that help restore self-worth, give people the right to work, to make decisions. In short, offer people the same kind of inclusion the rest of us take for granted. People, *all* people, need to fulfil a useful role in society. When people are excluded, their potential denied, we cannot possibly expect them to be whole.

The authors are not scientists, have neither the knowledge nor the resources to prove some of our beliefs. But we know what we have seen. And we have seen that the best outcomes happen when people – regardless of diagnosis – are valued.

There are scores of disorders listed in the psychiatric manuals. Disorders that reduce people to symptoms, categories, labels. But when it comes right down to it, there really are only eight kinds of people who suffer from issues of mental health. Someone's husband, father, brother, or son; someone's mother, daughter, sister, or wife.

KATHERINE'S STORY

I've heard too many times from friends and others that schizo-phrenia means split personality. These comments really hurt me. But what used to hurt me more was that I would remain silent. I did not try to defend people who have schizophrenia. This made me angry with myself. But I've gotten better at defending people who have schizophrenia after a long period of living with the illness. Schizophrenia may mean a person is split from reality. But schizophrenia has nothing to do with personalities.

I have heard other negative comments about those who have schizophrenia. The media will say, "A schizophrenic killed some-one today." But they never say, "A diabetic killed someone today." Because the media only reports negative views on people who have schizophrenia, the general population is led to believe that all people who have schizophrenia are criminals, murder-ers, or some sort of evil monsters. The media is so efficient in portraying these negative views that when I was first diagnosed with schizophrenia I really believed that one day I would turn into an axe murderer or worse.

When I first went to a psychiatrist, at sixteen years old, he told me I was just suffering from an identity crisis. But I went back to him a second time. In his office were old heat radiators that made a strange noise, and I thought there was a tape recorder behind the doctor's chair. Paranoia set in, and I was diagnosed with schizophrenia a short time later by this same doctor. I'm twenty-seven now, so I have lived with the illness for eleven years.

My childhood and early adolescence were happy times. My family has always been very supportive. Right from the start of my illness, my parents were really understanding. If it were not for my parents, I'd have been dead by now.

Schizophrenia turned my life upside down. My parents noticed I was withdrawn and not myself. They noticed I worried more. I could not answer the phone or doorbell, because I was afraid that whoever I talked to would be mad at me or would want to harm me in some way. I couldn't listen to the television or radio either, because they would also trigger a worry. My room seemed to be the place where I felt safest. I spent most of my time there. Sleep seemed to be the only thing that could briefly stop my anxiety, paranoia, and delusions.

I ended up missing half my Grade 11 and Grade 12 years. I would be sick for two weeks, and then well for two weeks. Just as I was getting caught up, I would get sick again. It was a vicious cycle, and it was very frustrating. I don't know how I graduated.

Along with paranoia and anxiety, another symptom of mine is having what I call DLTs. DLTs stand for "delusional thinkings." And delusions are false beliefs. I find with my delusions that sometimes 50% of me believes the delusion is reality and 50% of me believes the delusion is false. But this percentage fluctuates a lot. Most of the time at least 10% of me believes the delusion to be false.

Once, I thought I was getting messages from licence plates. A license plate, for example, would read CIN 200. I thought this meant I had to drive to the Cinnamon's restaurant and wait for someone who would tell me the truth about my past. I would wait in various restaurants depending on what a licence plate said. Sometimes I would wait for hours. Of course no one came to meet me.

At times I have thought I was an angel who had the ability to heal people with prayers. Sometimes I have also thought I could predict the future. Psychiatrists have diagnosed me with everything: schizoaffective disorder, manic depression, and so on. Most of these mental illnesses are closely related, so it is often hard for doctors to diagnose someone. My latest diagnosis is schizophrenia. I do believe I have a mild form of schizophrenia.

Over the years I've found medications have worked for me for a short time and then suddenly don't work any longer. It is a trial-and-error process. Today, I still experience some delusions and depression. Sometimes my delusions occupy my mind for days or weeks. I try to keep busy so I don't think so much about them. But the DLTs I experience now are not as bad as they used to be, even though some of them are the same.

There was only one time when I had an auditory hallucination. I was on a train ride in Scotland and a voice told me I was going to bite my tongue. I would say no, the voice would say yes. We went back and forth, saying no and yes, for about thirty minutes. I guess I won the argument, because I did not bite my tongue. The only visual hallucination I've experienced was seeing red paint on my forehead. It looked like an aboriginal design. I didn't see it in the mirror for very long. I still don't know what to make of that.

Until recently, I hadn't told friends I've known for over ten years that I have schizophrenia. To my surprise they did not treat me any differently, and I'm still friends with them. It really bothered me that I had kept it a secret. I felt like I was lying to my friends. Originally I told them I had a mysterious disease from the time I visited Africa in 1988 when I was sixteen. My friends believed that story for the longest time.

I am really glad I'm a part of the Partnership Program,* educating various people about schizophrenia. Most of the time I feel like I'm an outsider looking in. With the Partnership Program, I feel like I have a place in society, that I fit somewhere. It is a good feeling.

---

* The Partnership Program, run by the Schizophrenia societies of Alberta and Saskatchewan, introduces high school students to young people with schizophrenia, who talk about their lives. Katherine (a pseudonym) is one of the participants.

During my eleven years of having schizophrenia I have done a lot of volunteer work, and I have also held full-time summer jobs. I graduated in 1997 with a B.A. in English. I'm presently in my third year of a B.A. in social work. My goal is to become a psychiatrist. Many people say that becoming a doctor is unrealistic. But I'm an optimistic person. I find I need challenges and obstacles in my life to survive. My biggest obstacle has been schizophrenia, and I've somewhat overcome that.

CHAPTER FOUR

What *Is* Mental Disorder?

Madness has been and remains an elusive thing.
                    – Roy Porter, medical historian

Ask a hundred Canadians this question – What is mental disorder? – and you'll likely get a hundred different answers. And a lot of them will be just plain wrong. A character flaw, laziness, lack of discipline, the devil at work; such answers still repeatedly pop up in public surveys.

We'll talk more about stigma in Chapter 11. For now, let's just agree that these answers clearly *are* wrong. What we're interested in here are the right answers. We want scientific proof, concrete evidence, about what mental disorder is and where it comes from. So we turn to modern science – to the researchers of psychiatry, psychology, and social science who devote their careers to the subject.

The curious thing is, here, too, you won't find much of a consensus. Even within disciplines, there is plenty of debate. Truth is, despite huge advances in technology and treatment, *no one* really knows what happens, in the mind or the brain, when mental disorder strikes. We're still a long way from understanding the dynamics of any one disorder, let alone the broader concept of disorder itself.

Today, we have plenty of theories, and research flowing from them. But they remain just that – theories, or best guesses. In this chapter, we'll talk about some of those best guesses. They're important not just to researchers, but to consumers and family members as well. History has shown that as our notions of disorder shift, so does the treatment we receive.

Those notions can be divided into two basic parts: what *counts* as disorder, and what *causes* it.

WHAT COUNTS?

Diagnosis is the cornerstone of all medicine. And diagnosis depends upon classification. There are any number of physical diseases and disorders, each with an assigned name. Something goes wrong with some part of the body, and the doctor knows just what to call it.

Psychiatrists follow this medical model; they think of each mental disorder as a separate pathological entity, just like diabetes or tuberculosis. The problem is, we know a lot more about physical disorders than mental ones. Doctors have a good idea of what happens in the pancreas or the lungs when diabetes or tuberculosis strikes. But the mind is far more complex, and nailing down the true nature of its disorders is much harder to do.

How, then, do doctors go about diagnosing mental disorder? What tools do they use to define, for example, schizophrenia?

"We're relying on a person's personal experience of something and how they describe it to us, as a diagnostician, and those are not very reliable ways," says Dr. Mary Seeman, a Canadian authority on schizophrenia. "But that's all we have to go on. We don't have anything else, so that's how we define this nebulous illness, and there's no blood test, there's no X-ray. There's really nothing, other than symptoms."

Symptoms – the pain or problem or experience you describe to your doctor – are obviously important in physical illness too. But in psychiatry, they play a much more pivotal role.

The book that North American psychiatrists use for diagnosis is called the *Diagnostic and Statistical Manual of Mental Disorders* (or DSM), now in its fourth edition. In the world of psychiatry, the DSM defines what counts as disorder. Produced by the American Psychiatric Association, it lists scores of different conditions, each defined by a set of symptoms.

The approach is "descriptive"; the manual defines disorders by what they look like, with no need to understand what causes them. That's because psychiatrists don't *know* what causes most disorders.

"What is the cause of something like erotomania, the delusional belief that someone else is in love with you?" University of Toronto professor Edward Shorter writes in his book *A History of Psychiatry*. "Nobody knows. Psychiatric illness has tended therefore to be classified on the basis of symptoms rather than causes, which is where the rest of medicine was in the nineteenth century."

Most psychiatrists would argue that a symptom-based classification system is better than none at all. Better because it gives clinicians and researchers a common language, so that when they talk about "schizophrenia," everyone knows what the term describes. Better, too, because different treatments can be tailored for different disorders; lithium, for example, is considered an effective treatment for bipolar disorder but not for schizophrenia.

Before the DSM became popular, psychiatrists were accused of making random diagnoses. According to one old joke, if you put a hundred psychiatrists in a room with a patient you'll wind up with a hundred and one diagnoses. (The last one comes from the patient.) That joke no longer applies. While misdiagnosis is still a problem, there's far more consensus than in the past, because psychiatrists now use a common set of criteria.

But those criteria don't tell us much about the disorders themselves. They provide labels attached to lists of symptoms. And not much else. As one critic puts it, "The nature of the 'thing' described remains entirely obscure." Does the diagnosis represent an actual illness, caused by some physiological pathology? Does it represent an adaptation – a behavioural or emotional response – to life experiences? Or is it some combination of these things? Nobody knows for sure. (For this reason, we've chosen to use the term mental *disorder* instead of *illness* in this book.)

The longer the labels are used – and they've been around for several decades now – the greater the risk that we'll put too much stock in them.

"If you don't have the labels it's a mess, because you don't have a language," says Dr. John Strauss, a professor emeritus at Yale Medical School, and a pre-eminent thinker in the field. "And if you do have the labels there's a danger of believing too much in them. I don't have any problem with the current labels, but I wish people weren't so confident that they knew what they meant."

You might wonder how psychiatrists come up with these labels. How do diagnoses make it on to the pages of the DSM? This, too, is controversial. Task forces and work groups get together and agree upon names and matching symptoms. In effect, they *create* categories of disorder by consensus – something other fields of medicine don't do.

"I don't believe the gastroenterologists have task forces to decide whether constipation and pylorospasm should be listed as diseases or not," an objecting member of one DSM task force stated.

The task-force members have tried to base their decisions on "empirical evidence." They want the process to be as scientific as possible. But definitions based on symptoms – especially ones that involve behaviour, personality, thoughts, and feelings – are bound to be subjective. What one culture deems normal, another might call abnormal. What one individual considers to be illness might through different eyes look like mere eccentricity. In North America alone, our notions of what counts as mental disorder have changed dramatically over the past century.

"Our concepts of what mental illnesses are are so elastic," says Dr. Morton Beiser, vice-chair of research at the University of Toronto's Department of Psychiatry. "It's not just a question of medical disorders or psychiatric disorders; it's also a question of what does society define as . . . within the purview of mental illness."

Some critics argue our concepts are *so* elastic they're meaningless. The antipsychiatry movement – some of its most vocal members being renegade psychiatrists – claims that mental disorder is a purely social construct, not part of medicine at all.

As the well-known critic Thomas Szasz puts it in his book *The Myth of Mental Illness*, physical illnesses look the same the world over. "But this is emphatically not true for the phenomenology of so-called mental illness, whose manifestations depend upon and vary with the educational, economic, religious, social and political character of the individual and the society in which it occurs."

Homosexuality is a good example. Once listed as a mental disorder, task-force members voted to drop it from the DSM in 1973, after intense lobbying from gay-rights groups. "It was less clear that this was a scientific issue than it was, at least in part, a political one," Dr. Mitchell Wilson wrote in the *American Journal of Psychiatry*.

Other disorders have disappeared from the list as medical advances are made. Epilepsy was listed in early versions of the DSM. It's now been dropped, moved to the domain of neurology. The same has happened with other disorders once considered psychiatric.

"Historically, once etiology [the cause] is known, a disease stops being 'psychiatric,'" Drs. Daniel Goodwin and Samuel Guze write in their book *Psychiatric Diagnosis*. "Vitamins were discovered, whereupon vitamin-deficiency psychiatric disorders no longer were treated by psychiatrists. The spirochete was found, then penicillin, and neurosyphilis, once a major psychiatric disorder, became one more infection treated by nonpsychiatrists."

While some disorders have been dropped, many others have been added, all with causes unknown or unstated. In fact, the DSM has grown significantly. With each new edition; the list of what counts as disorder gets ever longer. Why is this happening? Is science providing more insights into the many ways the mind becomes disordered? Or are psychiatrists lowering the threshold, pathologizing behaviours even slightly removed from "normal"?

It's a question critics often ask. A scathing review of the latest edition of the DSM, appearing in *Harper's Magazine*, raised questions about psychiatrists' motives. "Here, on a staggering scale, are gathered together all the known mental disturbances of humankind," writes L.J. Davis, "the illnesses of mind and spirit that cry out for the therapeutic touch of – are you ready for this? – the very people who first wrote the book." The article notes that the more disorders listed, the more doctors' billing opportunities, too.

You'd probably be surprised to read some of what counts as disorder in the DSM. Alongside long-standing and widely recognized disorders like depression or anorexia nervosa, you'll find such conditions as Stuttering, Mathematics Disorder, Caffeine Intoxication, Nicotine Dependence, Pain Disorder, Sleep Disorder – Jet Lag Type. New to the fourth edition is Feeding Disorder of Infancy or Early Childhood, for children who don't eat adequately or gain weight. Also Substance-induced Sexual Dysfunction, for adults whose sexual problems are "fully explained by substance abuse."

As the *Harper's* article notes: "Hangnails seem to have avoided the amoeba's kiss, and the common cold is momentarily safe (unless it is accompanied by pain) but precious little else is."

One important proviso is that the disorders listed in the DSM generally include a "clinical significance" criterion.

The symptoms have to cause "clinically significant distress or impairment in social, occupational, or other important areas of functioning." That means, if your coffee consumption doesn't bother you, it doesn't count as a disorder. In clinical terms, the DSM authors were trying to reduce so-called "false positives" – a diagnosis given for unusual but not pathological behaviour.

Even so, the authors of *Psychiatric Diagnosis* – both well-known psychiatrists – have raised a cautionary flag about the vast majority of DSM diagnoses. "In our view there are only about a dozen diagnostic entities in adult psychiatry that have been sufficiently studied to be useful." The authors argue that only these twelve – which include affective, schizophrenic, panic, phobic, and eating disorders – "can be defined explicitly, and have a more or less predictable course."

These are the disorders most of us will have heard of. If you haven't experienced depression or mania, panic attacks or phobia, you probably know someone who has. And you'd immediately recognize the symptoms listed in the DSM.

Perhaps the most controversial diagnoses in the DSM fall under the category of "personality disorders." We all have personality traits – shyness, impulsiveness, and so on. These become labelled disorders when taken to an extreme. But how to decide what counts as extreme? Where's the line between normal and abnormal when you're talking about personality? Here's a description of one group of personality disorders in a textbook for clinicians called *DSM-IV Made Easy*: "People with the Cluster B disorders tend to be dramatic, emotional, and attention-seeking; their moods are labile and often shallow. They often have intense interpersonal conflicts." That might sound like any number of people you know.

Again, there's a requirement of significant distress or impairment. The DSM states that personality disorders must also involve "an enduring pattern of inner experience and behavior that deviates markedly from the expectations of the individual's culture." But still, "enduring" or "markedly" are subjective words. As is "culture."

Some women's groups have taken exception to one diagnosis in particular: borderline personality disorder (BPD).
It's diagnosed more often in women, and often women who've
been physically or sexually abused. The symptoms include
recurrent suicidal or self-mutilating behaviour, feelings of
emptiness, and frantic efforts to avoid abandonment. Do these
symptoms represent pathology . . . or just an understandable
response to trauma?

"I think that borderline personality can be dismantled,"
says Dr. Brenda Toner, head of the women's mental health
program at the Centre for Addiction and Mental Health in
Toronto. "If you look at the behaviours that go into borderline personality, then I think it would be more helpful in terms
of describing what the person's going through rather than
putting a label on it. . . . I guess it's not 100% trauma but it's
a huge component."

Dr. Toner thinks BPD symptoms would be better defined,
and treated, as a form of Post-traumatic Stress Disorder.

Which kind of gets us back to where we started. We still
don't *really* know what causes something like BPD.

WHAT CAUSES DISORDER?

Many great minds have tried to answer this question. And many
of them have looked to the body. In ancient Greece, Hippocrates
thought melancholia (his word for what we now call depression)
was caused by an accumulation of black bile. Hysteria was
thought to originate in the womb (or *hyster*), so only women
could get it. Later theories pointed to the heart producing
vapours that condensed in the brain. The colon harbouring
toxins. The nervous system itself becoming agitated, causing
nervous states. Treatments were also physical: laxatives, blood-
letting, cold baths, spa treatments. As Roy Porter writes in his
book *A Social History of Madness*, "Treating the body was
intended to have its impact on the mind as well."

Another approach that's reappeared throughout history
was to think of madness as a kind of curse. So we had the

medieval belief in witches' hexes or satanic possessions. The cure was exorcism, and incantations.

It's easy to laugh at these old ideas. But who's to say that centuries from now our own notions of disorder won't seem just as ludicrous? Researchers say that today's approaches are rooted firmly in science. But psychiatry is a young science. Some would even argue it isn't a science at all.

Today, most researchers agree that no one thing causes disorder. Whatever the final answer is, it's unlikely to be quite so simple.

"There's nothing in our existence that's caused by a single thing," says Dr. Peter Liddle, a prominent schizophrenia researcher and head of psychiatry at the University of British Columbia. "If a fire breaks out in a building, what caused the fire? The fact that somebody put a hot object in touch with a flammable object? The fact there was oxygen in the air? The fact that somebody didn't check the security of the building? There are actually many, many different things that have to occur before a fire can break out in a building."

In recognition of this complexity, the word now widely used to describe mental disorder is "biopsychosocial." It acknowledges that biological, psychological, and social elements all play a role in creating (and treating) mental disorder. That sounds great on paper, but in practice it's not so easily applied, because we still don't know quite *how* these elements intertwine.

"That's another place where being able to accept a fair amount of ignorance would be really helpful," says Dr. Strauss when asked about the term. "It's not like you just add them all together. We don't really understand, I think, how the bio, the psycho, and the social interact."

This is where "biopsychosocial" can become a bit of a hollow shell. Although psychiatrists will tell you that none of the elements should be overlooked, they're all bound to emphasize one over another. As Dr. Beiser says, "Everybody has their own pet view of what's really going to turn out to be important."

And what they think is most important is what they'll focus on in research. In practice, those differing approaches have tended to break down into biological or psychosocial. Heredity or environment. Nature or nurture. The age-old debate is still alive and well today.

"Psychiatry has always been torn between two visions of mental illness," Dr. Shorter writes in *A History of Psychiatry*. "One vision stresses the neurosciences, with their interest in brain chemistry, brain anatomy, and medication, seeing the origin of psychic distress in the biology of the cerebral cortex. The other vision stresses the psychosocial side of patients' lives, attributing their symptoms to social problems or past personal stresses, to which people may adjust imperfectly."

This is where culture comes into play. Thirty years ago, psychoanalysis was "in," and the focus was on early-childhood experiences. Today, biological research is dominant. In our quick-fix world, psychiatric drugs have become a multi-billion dollar business, with a pill for every problem.

"There is a kind of sociology of science," Dr. Beiser says. "In the sixties and seventies, the social model was the paramount model, and it was very hard to get funding to do research in genetics. Everybody was putting their money on social factors. . . . Now it's biology. It's neurochemistry, it's brain imaging, it's genetics. No question that's getting the most play."

This emphasis has spilled over into treatment: more on pharmacology, less on psychological or social solutions. And it's spilled over into popular consciousness, too. The media have jumped on the biological bandwagon. Stories abound about the latest genetic breakthrough, the newest brain scan image, the next wonder drug. Major research institutes regularly trumpet new discoveries, even "proof," that various disorders have biochemical or genetic causes.

It's important, amidst all the hype, to stress that there is no final proof. Lots of tantalizing evidence is being accumulated, but it's still just pieces of a puzzle, not yet complete.

BRAIN SCANS

Some of the puzzle pieces come from new technologies. Scanners like PET (positron emission tomography) and MRI (magnetic resonance imaging) machines can take pictures of the brain, which researchers use to look for neurological differences between people diagnosed with disorders and people who aren't.

Sometimes, they look at the structure of the brain. One 1990 study that got a lot of attention compared sets of identical twins, where one adult twin was diagnosed with schizophrenia and the other not. They found the twins with schizophrenia had slightly smaller brains than their siblings. A couple of specific regions of the brain were also smaller. This was hailed as a major breakthrough, "proof" that schizophrenia was a brain disorder.

Some critics argue these studies have been conducted on patients who've taken neuroleptic drugs or received electroconvulsive therapy, and that it's these treatments – not the schizophrenia – that account for any differences. (Indeed, some brain scans of people with schizophrenia support this view; long-term use of antipsychotic drugs may be correlated with changes in brain structure.)

Other research has focused on chemical neurotransmitters in the brain, which help brain cells communicate with each other. There's a theory that these chemicals become disrupted, causing a disorder. An overactive dopamine system, for example, in schizophrenia. Low levels of serotonin in depression. Psychiatric drugs are formulated to act on those same systems, often relieving symptoms. But is this proof that chemical imbalances *cause* the disorders?

"That's, again, a broad generalization that's too early to make," says Dr. Jacques Bradwejn, a researcher and chairman of Psychiatry at the University of Ottawa. "You could say serotonin is disrupted in depression. Many people will respond to a drug that acts on serotonin. That doesn't mean we know exactly what the cause is."

In fact, we're only beginning to explore the brain's complex neural networks – how many chemicals are in there, and how they interact with one another. For now, we know very little.

"There is absolutely no evidence that 'biochemical imbalances' cause mental disorders," renowned neuroscientist Dr. Candace Pert told a convention of Ontario psychiatrists.

In recent years, thanks to a new machine called an FMRI (for functional magnetic resonance imaging), researchers have also been able to take pictures of the brain at work. They study the way the brain *functions*. Subjects lie inside the scanning machine, performing a prescribed task, and researchers observe patterns of activity – which parts of the brain "light up" or become active. Again, they're looking for differences between groups of people with a disorder and those without.

Dr. Liddle is especially interested in finding a pattern of activity characteristic of schizophrenia. "Maybe we're getting there," he says. "I wouldn't want to be too confident. But on the other hand I've been working for the past few years on looking at the way that co-ordination of activity between different brain areas occurs, and the way that the brain works as a coherent whole. And there are certain patterns that seem to be characteristic of schizophrenia."

The big question is, what do these patterns tell us about the disorder? The easy answer would be that there's some biological pathology of the brain that causes the disorder. People are born with a "schizophrenic brain," which acts in abnormal ways. Interestingly enough, Dr. Liddle doesn't reach this conclusion. The brain, he says, is not fixed but ever-changing, responding to stimuli – stresses, pleasures – and the tasks it's given.

"We know that a whole lot of social or psychological things actually change not only the functioning of the brain but the structure of the brain. We know that whenever you do anything, when you talk . . . or when you give someone a hug . . . these things represent things going on in the brain."

The environment helps *shape* the brain, affecting its growth and development over a lifespan. For example, research has shown measurable changes in the brain as a result of psycho-therapy. As one psychiatrist puts it, "There is a constant interplay between environmental factors and brain develop-ment." This concept of the brain as a highly responsive organ has been described as "plasticity" – and it's an area that has generated much enthusiasm in recent years.

In practice, brain scans may tell us as much about our life experiences as our biology. "We now know, for example, through neuroimaging, that the history of trauma actually influences brain activation," says Dr. Toner. "So even if you see differences in the brain, it doesn't necessarily mean that it's a biological difference. It could be caused by a chronic envi-ronmental stressor like a trauma."

In effect, then, we're back to the "which came first" ques-tion. Finding discrete patterns of activity might prove useful for clinicians – Dr. Liddle hopes it will help with diagnosis – but brain-imaging work still won't tell us whether schizophrenia, or any other mental disorder, is biological in origin. (In fact, Dr. Liddle and many other researchers now believe that "schizo-phrenia" may actually be several different disorders, with different causes, all now erroneously lumped under one label. That would help explain the vastly different courses it can take.)

GENETICS

It's extremely popular these days. Research institutions around the world are pouring money into DNA labs. So far, there's been no definitive proof, no replicated studies confirming a "depression gene" or an "anxiety gene." Critics say there never will be. But people working in the field believe it's just a matter of time.

One massive international effort, the Human Genome Project, promises to identify and locate every gene on our chromosomes by the year 2003. Advances in DNA techno-logies have made this possible. And it's thought the findings will have profound implications for our understanding of many mental disorders.

Genetic work itself is not new. In the past century, hundreds of studies have compared rates of disorder among twins, family members, and adopted children. These studies have generally found that schizophrenia, bipolar disorder, panic, and anxiety disorders tend to run in families.

In twin studies, researchers look at "concordance rates": how often *both* twins develop schizophrenia, for example. Identical twins have identical genes, and they have higher concordance rates than fraternal twins (who developed in the womb from two separate eggs rather than from one egg that split). The same is true for bipolar disorder. This suggests genes do play a role.

Research has also shown that children are more likely to be diagnosed with schizophrenia when one or both parents has been diagnosed. This holds true even when children are adopted out at an early age.

Dr. James Kennedy, a genetics researcher at Toronto's Centre for Addiction and Mental Health, calls these findings "very, very strong evidence that a major portion of the risk for the more severe psychiatric disorders is inherited."

Of course, not everybody in a family will wind up with a diagnosis. Even between identical twins, the concordance rate is never 100%. And there are a couple of theories about why that might be. Maybe several genes are involved in any one disorder.

"Maybe three genes come together to cause schizophrenia, for example," says Dr. Kennedy. "So grandfather might have had all three, and he passed two to his son. So his son didn't have enough of the genetic load to get the disorder. But then his son married a woman who unfortunately had this third gene, and three of their kids would be just fine but one of them would have the same disorder that grandpa had, because those three bad genes came together again."

Another important point – and even the most enthusiastic genetics researchers would agree – is that biology can't explain everything. Even if specific genes are one day linked to specific disorders, environment will still play a role. Researchers now talk about a genetic *vulnerability*.

"We all carry many, many dormant genes within us that still have to get turned on somehow," says Dr. Seeman. "And that's where the environment comes in."

In other words, life events and stressors are the triggers that can turn vulnerability into disorder. "You could use the analogy of a broken leg," says John Allen, a researcher and associate professor of psychology at the University of Arizona. "We all have the potential for a broken leg. Some have a stronger potential than others, because they have weaker bones. But it's not until you slip on the curb that you actually break your leg."

These triggers seem to be different for different people. Here's where psychological and social factors come into play – factors that are too easily forgotten in the rush for biological answers. And yet, for many consumers, the psychological and social elements clearly matter most.

ENVIRONMENT

It's obvious, but not often stated: what happens to us in our daily lives is bound to affect how we think and feel. Psychiatrists who specialize in psychotherapy observe this as they work with clients.

"I can comfortably state that I have never seen a patient who experienced a depression for no reason whatsoever," one clinical psychiatrist wrote in a letter published in the *National Post* newspaper. "From my perspective, those psychiatrists who speak of such 'endogenous' depressions just did not explore their patients' lives deeply enough."

Research confirms that psychological and social factors *do* play a role. As with biological factors, they cannot fully predict whether any one person will develop a disorder. But when you look at larger numbers, you start to see trends: risk factors associated with higher rates of disorder, and protective factors associated with lower rates.

"When you move to a high population level, you can really make some correlations," says David Cohen, a professor of social work at the University of Montreal. "Prosperity is associated with less distress. You can say that. There's very strong evidence for that."

In fact, income is one of the strongest predictors of health – including mental health – we've found. Poverty is a risk factor; wealth is a protective factor. That doesn't mean everyone who's poor develops mental health problems.

"There's things that intervene," Prof. Cohen continues. "We call them social supports: self-esteem, coping resources, social networks. Those things protect people from the stress of poverty."

Ironically, those social supports may be less available to people at lower income levels. Canadian research has shown, for example, that as income levels drop, rates of emotional and behavioural problems in children go up. It has also found that safe neighbourhoods, residential and school stability, and involvement in sports, recreation, and arts activities reduce the risk of childhood emotional problems.

So if you add enough social risk factors together, people become more vulnerable. The same applies for psychological factors, many of which go right back to childhood. As we've seen in Chapter 3, the Ontario Mental Health Survey found a strong link between serious physical or sexual abuse in childhood and mental disorder in adult life.

That finding comes as no surprise to Pat Fisher, a trauma specialist. In her recent study of in-patients at Riverview Hospital, a psychiatric facility in Vancouver, 58% of the women she surveyed revealed a history of childhood trauma.

"This group had much higher proportions of not only childhood sexual abuse and physical abuse," Dr. Fisher says, "but they also had much higher levels of disruptions in care, multiple caregivers, parental neglect, family violence, and on and on. So there's just this whole litany of risk factors, and of assaults on self."

Again, there's no straight cause-and-effect. Not all the women surveyed had a trauma history. And clearly, not everyone who experiences abuse develops a disorder. Dr. Fisher believes genetic vulnerability has a role to play, too. "On the one hand, you've got the vulnerability. And that's a fixed factor. And then, when you lay the stresses on top of that, the risks for that vulnerability to be expressed go up."

Even when there is no abuse, there can be risk factors in the family. Family dysfunction and inconsistent or negative parenting patterns can have an effect. If a parent is depressed, for example, the risk of a child developing emotional or behavioural problems goes up.

A recent Health Canada report emphasizes the importance of young children forming a "secure attachment" with a parent, based on a loving, secure relationship. "Infants . . . whose parents are unable to form this attachment due to illness or stress are at higher risk for a number of behavioural, social and cognitive problems in later life."

Called *Toward a Healthy Future*, the report also cites recent studies in neurobiology that suggest early experiences can actually affect how the brain is wired. Neglect or abuse "may produce wiring patterns in the brain that can lead to heightened sensitivity to stimuli and to negative and abnormal behaviour in childhood and adulthood. In other words, the environment around an infant has a major influence on the brain's development and subsequently on a person's capacity for control over intense feelings, including anxiety and aggression."

All of which suggests that nature and nurture are ultimately inseparable. Where does one begin and the other end? How can this even be determined?

"When is it that a certain kind of early childhood experience has certain kinds of effects on the brain?" Dr. Strauss asks. "When is it that a certain genetic makeup influences how early childhood effects have a certain influence on the brain? It's incredibly complicated, I think."

Nonetheless, the nature-versus-nurture debate remains a heated one. For some people the idea that their genes or brain chemistry are somehow defective is morally offensive, and implies that they're lesser human beings. For other people, a biological explanation brings immense relief. And that includes many parents, who object to the notion that they may be to blame for their child's disorder.

In the end, we each must find our own answer to the question "What is mental disorder?" And there is good news in this inability of experts to answer the question for us. In the absence of definitive proof, every opinion is as valid as the next.

And that includes your own.

J E H A N ' S   S T O R Y *

Her name was Mariam. And she was drop dead gorgeous. She was tall, lithe, and had luxurious waist-length raven hair. My heart would pound and inch up to my vocal chords, choking off any sound I tried to make whenever she said "Hi!" Happiness or despair depended upon how much of her precious time she allocated to me. She ruled my world. We were both thirteen and she was my first crush. Although I wanted to proclaim my love for her to anyone who would listen, I felt ashamed and terrified of my feelings because I was not the opposite sex. So I kept Mariam locked up in the safety of my heart. Thus began my reign of shame and secrecy, which was to last for nineteen long years.

That same year, my family moved from Tanzania to Vancouver. My first years in Vancouver were hell. Although I was fluent in English, I had trouble understanding the Canadian accent and found it hard to keep up with the speed at which people spoke. I dreaded going to school. Some classmates would pepper me with spitballs almost on a daily basis. At lunchtime, no one would want to sit near a "Paki." After school, I would be spat

* This story was originally published in a slightly different form in the CMHA B.C. journal *Visions.* "Jehan" is a pseudonym. Reprinted by permission.

on, pushed, and called "Paki" and "Hindu." I couldn't understand such hostility. I would stare at my face in the mirror to see if I had some kind of defect.

In Grade 9 I fell in love with Anna. What luck and joy – not only was Anna white, she was a lesbian! This bubble burst, however, when some boys from our class caught us kissing. From then on, we were taunted unmercifully, and "Paki" was replaced with "Butch" and "Lesbo."

To make things worse, a friend of the family saw Anna and me in a "compromising position." My poor parents. I was racked with guilt and sadness for them. I felt that I had failed them.

My dad asked if I was a lesbian. I said, "Yes." He hugged me and made arrangements for me to see a psychiatrist. I felt so despondent and shameful. Not only had I committed a sin, but there was something wrong with me mentally. After a few sessions with me, the psychiatrist explained to my parents that I was a borderline lesbian. My parents hoped I would eventually fall on the "right" side of the border. Even I felt hopeful that I could be "cured"!

Unfortunately for them, and despite my best intentions, I fell in love with another woman. My parents abandoned the psychiatrist and turned to God, churning out prayers in a fever pitch. When the incense smoke cleared, I was secretly relieved to find I was still a lesbian. I reasoned that if God wouldn't intervene, then, just maybe, loving a woman wasn't a sin.

The woman I had fallen in love with was also a South Asian. Outwardly, Jehanara and I acted like friends, and my parents felt safe in their knowledge that there couldn't possibly be another South Asian lesbian on the planet! But a year after we graduated from high school, Jehanara did the "respectful" thing and got married.

When Jehanara decided not to see me anymore, I was heartbroken. I couldn't envision life without her. I felt too ashamed to even talk to anyone about it. At nineteen, it felt like my life was over. I contemplated killing myself, but the thought of my mom's pain and the possibility that my soul would never rest stopped me. Deep down I knew I could never change, and I didn't know whether that was good or bad.

My parents felt it was time I got married. Even I wanted relief from my life. Thus began the quest for a husband. My parents knew of a "good Muslim man" in England. Photos were exchanged, I liked what I saw, and went to England with the family to meet Hamid. After a few dates, he said he was in love with me. I told Hamid I wasn't sure about my feelings. He begged me to accept him. So I said, "Yes."

The marriage lasted four months. My parents were humiliated. I quit university and went to work in the family business in repentance.

As my thirtieth birthday loomed closer, I felt that my youth had gone, and that being a repeat offender I was past rehabilitation. As fate would have it, I started working in the heart of the gay district, where I couldn't help but notice the "homosexual" goings on. At first I was disgusted at the sheer audacity of "these people," kissing and holding hands in public and acting so normal. I had barricaded myself so tightly in the closet that I didn't see my hypocrisy. Gradually, I began to see them as individuals. My journey of self-acceptance had finally begun.

I had been aware of various lesbian coming-out support groups and finally summoned up the courage to go to one. In my eagerness to belong, I downplayed my "South Asianness," hoping that the all-white group would see me just as a lesbian. I couldn't bear the thought of being rejected by them. I was tolerated, but the camaraderie that I had so eagerly sought wasn't there. Only Alicia, the facilitator, seemed to treat me as an equal.

Alicia and I fell in love, and it felt truly liberating to be in a relationship with someone who was comfortable with her sexuality. I was able to find the strength to come out to my two closest friends and to my sisters, but I knew that to be completely true to myself, I still needed to come out to my parents.

Alicia was seeing a lesbian therapist and spoke glowingly about how she had helped her cope with difficult issues. Although wary of therapists because of my earlier experience with the psychiatrist, the prospect of a lesbian therapist was appealing.

My therapist was understanding, compassionate, and non-judgmental. What struck me most was the reassurance that I could talk about my sexuality without going into an automatic censor mode, or fearing that the listener might recoil in disgust. Gradually I felt strong enough to talk to my parents. On the day of "the talk," I felt none of the fear or shame that I thought I would. My dad's reaction was, "Well, if it's sex you want, then have it. But one day you will have to settle down with a man." My mom was surprisingly calm. I sensed that even though I had confirmed her worst fears about me, she felt relieved that it was finally out there.

Now in my late thirties and living openly with my current partner, I realize what a long journey I have been on. My family is slowly learning to accept us as a couple. I was thrilled the other day at how close to "home" my family and I had come when Dad personally invited my partner to a family barbecue.

CHAPTER FIVE

Schizo-what? – Getting Diagnosed

It's all in your head.

And that makes diagnosing a mental disorder a very tricky business.

Having someone else figure out what's going on in there, let alone *why* it's going on in there, is far from a perfect science. Some people report that they've had multiple diagnoses over time – and it wasn't until the correct diagnosis was made that an appropriate course of treatment could begin. One recent survey of U.S. consumers found it took people with bipolar affective disorder an average of *eight years* to receive a correct diagnosis. So it ain't foolproof.

Nor is it always welcome news; reactions to a diagnosis vary tremendously.

For some, being told you have a mental disorder, that you have a "mental illness," can be a shocking experience. Those words can strike us in a deeper, more frightening way than distressing news about our physical health. Lifelong perceptions, biases, prejudices can emerge with unexpected intensity. We may fear that we've somehow failed, that we'll never be the same, that people will judge us crazy.

Many people, particularly women who have suffered abuse or trauma, have told us of their strong objections to having their symptoms termed a disorder.

Conversely, receiving an accurate diagnosis can also bring tremendous relief. It offers an explanation for what may have been inexplicable thoughts or behaviours, reassures us we're not the only ones feeling this way. A diagnosis can also provide hope for improving the situation, because once we put the right name on this *thing*, we've got a road map to a myriad of treatment options.

As the previous chapter noted, diagnoses developed from a need for a common language, a frame of reference – and the need to collect statistical information. What was likely one of the first attempts to gather this information was the 1840 U.S. census, which tried to count how many people fell under the "idiocy/insanity" label. By the time the 1880 census rolled around, there were seven categories, including "mania" and "melancholia." That number has grown ever since.

While the *Diagnostic and Statistical Manual of Mental Disorders* (DSM) is regarded as psychiatry's "bible," there are plenty of atheists around. Critics argue that it pathologizes many aspects of normal human experience into categories of disorder. Even the DSM itself acknowledges that some of what it terms "disorders" would not be considered abnormal within certain ethnocultural or spiritual frameworks. (In some belief systems, it's perfectly normal to hear the voice of a dead relative – it's not necessarily a symptom of schizophrenia.)

Many psychiatrists from outside North America rely on a diagnostic manual developed by the World Health Organization. The *International Classification of Diseases* (ICD) contains similar, though not identical, classifications of mental disorder. Worldwide statistics, such as the Global Burden of Disease noted in Chapter 3, use the ICD as reference.

In North America, however, the DSM is the standard. It's worth repeating, however, that these terms are labels – they are a way of describing common clusters of symptoms that appear to be related. They are not names of concretely understood illnesses – and the manual itself does not use the word "illness."

The DSM also cautions against being used as a "cookbook," and rightly emphasizes that diagnosis should be made only by a qualified clinician. If you're interested in having a look at the book, most libraries – and certainly hospitals with a library – will have a copy.

In this chapter, we'll lay out some of the things psychiatrists look for when attempting to make a diagnosis. The purpose is to give you a *sense* of the symptoms commonly experienced, not to serve as a diagnostic tool of any kind. Do *not* assume, if you match symptoms in the following pages, that you have a disorder.

It's not as much fun as Letterman, but here's the "top ten" list of symptoms associated with common mental disorders. The first block falls under a category known as Mood Disorders. These include depression, bipolar affective disorder (manic depression), and seasonal affective disorder.

MOOD DISORDERS

Major Depression

As noted earlier, this mood disorder is – by one measure at least – the greatest disabler on earth. It is a very common diagnosis that directly, and indirectly, affects many millions of Canadians, young and old alike. And it can be pure hell.

When acute, depression is a crushing and overwhelming burden for any individual. It is far deeper, more paralyzing and debilitating, than merely having a case of the blues. Untreated, depression can be deadly. Up to 15% of all people with depression take their own lives (and up to 80% of people who suicide are depressed at the time of their death).

Most people suffering from depression report having at least five of the following symptoms and say they've lasted at least two weeks. To meet the criteria of a major depressive episode, the symptoms must be a departure from the way the person usually feels, must not have been triggered by the death of a loved one, and must be interfering with the person's everyday life. A clinician will also want to make sure that the symptoms have not been caused by a physical condition, medication, or substance abuse. Here are some of the typical ways you might feel if depressed.

- You feel sad or empty most of the time; a sadness or emptiness so overwhelming you feel powerless against it.
- You're sleeping too much or too little. Frequently, people in a severe depression can't even get out of bed.
- You're eating too much or too little. It's not uncommon to gain or lose a significant amount of weight during a depressive episode.
- You feel hopeless, worthless, and think the world would be better off without you.
- You feel guilty – even when there's no reason to be.
- Your body feels sluggish, you have no energy most of the time *or* you feel agitated and can't relax. Routine tasks like showering, shaving, or shopping can require considerable effort.
- You find it hard to think or concentrate; it's difficult to hold a thought.
- You're frequently thinking about suicide or death. Some people become fixated on dying. This is called "suicidal ideation."
- Nothing seems interesting or pleasurable any more; food can lose its taste, even the funniest movie can't bring a smile to your face. There is a total absence of joy in life.

Depression falls into a group of mood disorders also referred to as "affective disorders." Within that broad category are such variations on a theme as dysthymic disorder (low-level but chronic depression), substance-induced mood disorders, and others.

Postpartum depression is diagnosed when women develop depressive symptoms within four weeks of childbirth. Most new mothers experience the so-called "baby blues" – feelings of sadness, anxiety, and tearfulness in the week or so after a baby's birth. A smaller number – about 10% – develop the more severe and long-lasting symptoms of true depression. An even smaller number – as few as two in a thousand – suffer from a psychotic form of postpartum depression, experiencing delusions and hallucinations that may put them at risk of harming themselves or their baby. (Postpartum psychosis made front-page news in 2000 when a Toronto doctor jumped in front of a subway with her six-month-old baby in her arms; both died. Media reports emphasized her wealth and education, but her story proves the point that depression strikes people in every walk of life.)

The causes of postpartum depression are unclear, but may be related to hormonal changes. Women with a history of mood disorders, and women in an unhappy marriage, are at greater risk of developing the disorder. It's thought this type of depression is vastly underdiagnosed, in part because women fear being seen as bad mothers, even having their babies taken from them. This is unfortunate, because most women respond well to treatment, which consists of psychotherapy – especially interpersonal therapy – and/or antidepressants. If psychotic symptoms are present, hospitalization and antipsychotic medications may be required.

Depression is sometimes known as "*uni*polar affective disorder," meaning the person experiences just the deep and crushing lows. If, in addition to those desperate lows, they experience extraordinary highs, they may receive a diagnosis of "*bi*polar" affective disorder, previously known as manic depression.

The most common treatment for depression involves medication (antidepressants) and/or psychotherapy. Some studies indicate that psychotherapy is of equal benefit to drugs; other work suggests medication may be more effective. The vast majority of the literature indicates that the best results occur when both therapies are combined. There are, however, many alternatives that the evidence also supports as being useful – and which we'll cover later in the book.

Bipolar Affective Disorder

Bipolar affective disorder can be thought of as a roller coaster of mood. And, to stretch the analogy, it can be a helluva ride.

People with this disorder alternate, at varying speeds, between being low and being high. The lowest of the low is the depression just described. The highest of the high is something called a manic episode. Most people first go through a phase known as hypomania. This period could be described as "feeling good" – though it's more than that. It's an elevated, excitable, talkative phase during which a person feels quite energized. Your ability to think, to concentrate on the job, may even be enhanced during this period. Others may notice a change, but are unaware anything is wrong in its early stages. (This is true of many disorders.) Hypomania, in the typical sequence of events, is a prelude to mania – characterized by the following symptoms.

- You feel unbelievably, almost *indescribably*, good. Many have reported feeling "invincible." This elevated mood is a marked departure from "normal" mood and is accompanied by what feels like limitless energy.
- You need a lot less sleep. It's common for people in an acute manic phase to be unable to sleep at all – or only for an hour or two a night. That lack of sleep is believed to exacerbate manic symptoms and contribute to psychosis. (Even people *without* a mental disorder can become psychotic if deprived of sleep long enough.)
- You can become irritable or angry at the drop of a hat. Frequently, people in a manic or hypomanic stage can explode in anger at anyone who disagrees with or challenges their plans. This is, as with the other symptoms, a marked departure from the person's usual self.
- Your thoughts seem to jump around. You tend to talk very rapidly, and often feel that you can't stop talking. Its almost like you're being *forced* to speak. Clinically, these symptoms are known as "flight of ideas" and "pressure of speech." You've just gotta talk and talk and talk . . .

- You may spend far beyond your means, sometimes on very goofy things. A hallmark of a "classic" manic episode is a wild spending spree or unrealistic and grandiose business plan.
- Similarly, you might think you are unusually talented or gifted. Religious beliefs can intensify beyond all proportion. It is not uncommon for you to believe you are on a mission from God, even that you *are* God, or a person of great influence or importance. These are examples of psychotic thinking, where the person loses touch with reality.
- You lack inhibitions. Few people in the grip of mania have the ability to foresee the consequences of their actions. You may engage in indiscriminate sexual behaviour without a thought as to the ramifications.
- You lack insight. Despite all evidence to the contrary, you may be unable to see that your actions are inappropriate, irrational, or reckless. This is one of the bugaboos of the disorder – and a source of tremendous frustration for families and loved ones who can see something is seriously wrong.
- The symptoms haven't been caused by medication, substance use, or anything else you've been taking.
- The behaviour must be interfering with your life – and it almost always does.

The subjective experience of mania varies widely. Many recall it as the best they've felt in their lives; some have found it frightening. Still others believe it was a profound spiritual experience and reject any suggestion that a disorder was involved at all.

There are various forms of bipolar disorder. What's just been described, the classic depression and mania, is referred to as Bipolar I Disorder. If the person has depression accompanied by hypomania, but doesn't experience a manic episode, it's called Bipolar II. Some people, "rapid cyclers," can alternate between the crushing lows and electrifying highs within a very short period of time. There's also something known as "cyclothymia," where the highs aren't as high and the lows aren't as low, but the peaks and dips are nonetheless greater than other people experience in day-to-day life. Many people diagnosed with bipolar affective disorder have long periods – even years – of stability between episodes.

Depending on severity, bipolar disorder – in fact, all mood disorders – is not necessarily career-limiting. The late Pierre Péladeau, head of the gigantic Quebecor publishing firm, lived with ups and downs throughout his professional career. And he was in good company. A cover story in the March 1996 issue of *Canadian Business* labelled the disorder "The CEO's Disease," because many high-profile businesspeople share the diagnosis. One article noting similar accomplishments labelled such people "manic-impressives."

One website – <http://www.frii.com/~parrot/living.html> – lists successful folks who have publicly admitted experiencing either major depression or manic depression. While that's encouraging, don't forget that these disorders can also be terribly destructive – and some find them so disabling they are unable to work, let alone be creative.

A note of caution here. Some people with no previous history of this disorder have had a manic episode triggered by antidepressants. In other words, the medication that was supposed to lift you from a depression actually catapults you into the stratosphere. Those taking antidepressants who notice themselves feeling far more happy or energetic than usual should consult their physician.

One person we interviewed reported that his only two manic episodes occurred immediately following operations that required general anaesthetic. Others have experienced symptoms of mania following electroconvulsive therapy. Immense stress can trigger a manic episode, though some people seem to slide into mania for no discernible reason. There is a high rate, with this diagnosis, of alcohol abuse.

Treatment usually involves a combination of medication and psychotherapy. The pharmacological end of things generally involves a mood stabilizer such as lithium, sometimes in combination with an antidepressant.

Seasonal Affective Disorder (SAD)

Fall approaches. The leaves change to a golden amber, the sunsets take on a warm red hue, the days start getting shorter.

And you start feeling like poop.

Seasonal affective disorder is often referred to as SAD. It's an appropriate acronym, because that's how you feel. All of us can get moody on dark and stormy nights, but for people with this diagnosis, it's very different. When fall and winter approach, so does depression.

But, hey, most people wind down during winter, right? Well, yeah. As many as one in two Canadians will report some changes in mood, energy, and appetite across seasons. Those who suffer from SAD, however, experience those changes in a far more pronounced way. And though less than 5% of Canadians meet the criteria for a SAD diagnosis, that's still a lot of people.

In some ways, we shouldn't be surprised. Several studies have shown that people are more prone to the disorder in northern latitudes – though this correlation does not always hold true (Iceland, for example, has a relatively low incidence of SAD). What is consistent is that about 80% of sufferers are women between the ages of eighteen and forty-five. And some of their symptoms – strong cravings for carbohydrates and pronounced weight gain during fall and winter months – are atypical of most depressions. Many people with the disorder report being extremely fatigued; more than one has compared the experience to "hibernation."

To receive a diagnosis of SAD, a clinician will want to ensure there aren't other seasonal psycho-social stressors that could have triggered the depressive symptoms. Some people, for example, might regularly be unemployed during the fall and winter. Others might have annoying and unwanted relatives who come and stay for the holidays. These kinds of factors must be considered.

Diagnosticians will also explore the person's lifetime pattern of episodes. They'll be looking for clear evidence that depressions are far more likely to occur in the fall and winter than at other times of the year. If that seasonal/non-seasonal ratio is at least three to one, there's a strong case for SAD.

The first line of treatment for SAD is light therapy. This involves daily exposure to an artificial light source that mimics the sun's rays but provides ultraviolet protection. This seems to help in more than half of cases. Quite often, that treatment is supplemented with tryptophan, an amino acid. Generally, it's only when symptoms fail to respond to these efforts that an antidepressant is prescribed.

People with the disorder often suffer for years, wrongly assuming that their seasonal depressions are just a regular part of life. It doesn't have to be that way.

ANXIETY DISORDERS

Anxiety disorders are *the* most commonly reported mental health problem. In the Ontario Mental Health Supplement, 16% of all women and 9% of men reported anxiety-related symptoms during the previous twelve months – symptoms serious enough to interfere with many aspects of their daily lives.

And that, again, is the key in defining the disorder. Most of us get uptight when there are troubles at work, might get a shiver up our spine at finding a spider in the shower. That's normal; such anxieties are a part of life. For someone with an anxiety disorder, however, it's almost like these responses are being boosted by an amplifier with the volume cranked up. In these cases, the phrase "worried sick" can be literal.

The DSM lists several types of anxiety disorders; we'll touch on a few.

Generalized Anxiety Disorder

Worry, worry, worry. There are some people who just can't seem to stop. Of course, all of us fret over things. But if the worrying goes on and on and on, it could be time to take a look. Generalized anxiety disorder is a fairly common diagnosis, and many of us will relate to the symptoms. Fewer of us, however, will have experienced them over extended time frames. Here's what clinicians look for.

- You feel anxious or worried most of the time for a period of at least six months. These feelings must be out of proportion with the real-life circumstances that have prompted them.
- You can't seem to *control* the worry. No matter what steps you take to reduce the worry, it just keeps popping back into your head.
- The worry or anxiety seems to make you restless or on edge; exhausted after minor tasks; tense (including physical tension, tight muscles); have difficulty sleeping; have difficulty concentrating; irritable.
- The worry, anxiety, or symptoms must be serious enough to significantly interfere with aspects of your daily life, including your job or social life.

Treatment for generalized anxiety disorder has traditionally relied on either anti-anxiety medication (anxiolytics), psychotherapy, or both. In recent years it's been more widely acknowledged that some of these medications have addictive qualities. Some people, in fact, find that getting off the medication can lead to periods of anxiety even greater than was previously experienced.

There's good evidence that cognitive-behavioural therapy – which attempts to "short-circuit" faulty modes of thinking – is an effective treatment. The technique helps people realize that the level of anxiety was disproportionate, and it teaches techniques to nip it in the bud. Relaxation exercises can also be an effective tool in overcoming anxiety.

Panic Disorder

The words of poet Percy Bysshe Shelley have been around far longer than the words of the DSM, so it's interesting to consider these lines, taken from *The Indian Serenade*:

O lift me from the grass!
I die! I faint! I fail!
. . .
My cheek is cold and white, alas!
My heart beats loud and fast.

This almost exactly describes the sensations of a panic attack. It's an appropriate label, given the speed and power with which the physical symptoms envelop the person. So strong are the symptoms that many people have gone to hospital, repeatedly, convinced they may be on the verge of death.

Panic attacks are a graphic illustration of how our emotional and physical states can be virtually indistinguishable. Those with panic disorder frequently report many of the following symptoms occurring simultaneously.

- Your heart starts pounding, palpitating. People often say, "It felt like my heart would explode."
- You have difficulty breathing. It feels like there's a weight on your chest, that you're being smothered or choked. This can be so severe you feel almost paralyzed.
- You might have chest pains, as if you're having a heart attack.
- You can experience severe abdominal cramps or other gastrointestinal trouble. Often, these physical symptoms are reported to a family practitioner with neither the sufferer nor the physician realizing there may be a psychological root to the problem.
- You might start to tremble, shake, sweat.
- You might feel unsteady on your feet, dizzy, or faint.
- You can feel chilled or experience a hot flash.
- It might feel like you're "losing it" or "going crazy."
- You can experience overpowering dread; a fear that you're dying.

Remember, lots of people can experience feelings of panic. Your heart might pound before you board a flight, you may have butterflies before your guests arrive for a dinner party, get sweaty palms in a job interview. That's normal. But if you experience them frequently, simultaneously, and worry about future attacks, it's likely worth having a good physical and discussing it with your family doctor. Recent research has linked panic attacks with a heart condition known as mitral valve prolapse. In those cases, it may well *not* be in your head.

Treatment for panic attack should always include a good physical, to rule out any underlying arrhythmia (an irregular heartbeat). Anxiolytics (anti-anxiety medications) can be used in conjunction with psychotherapy, although a recent review of data by the Canadian Psychiatric Association (CPA) found that cognitive-behavioural therapy (CBT) is very effective on its own.

"Across a wide range of studies," reads the CPA synopsis, "an average of 85% of patients treated with CBT are panic-free at post-treatment, and 88% are panic-free at follow-up."

CBT is described on page 160.

Simple Phobia

A woman we know has a thing about snakes – she doesn't just dislike them, she's scared to death of 'em. In her case, the fear comes from a very unpleasant childhood experience: she was chased by a group of boys who shoved one down her shirt. It left her, as an adult, with a much-heightened fear of the reptiles – even ones she knows are harmless. If an innocent garter snake happens to slither too close, she is stricken with panic, a response she knows is disproportionate, but nonetheless cannot control. It's way beyond feeling simply nervous or squeamish.

Phobias are like that, though not all have their origins with snakes. Some people's responses are triggered by the sight of blood, getting on a plane . . . any number of objects or situations. These triggers provoke an *immediate* response, often a full panic attack. In all cases (except with some young children), people with the disorder *know* that their response is excessive yet are still incapacitated by it. Often, these folks will take extraordinary steps to avoid these triggers. For example, a businessman with a phobia about flights might decide to take the train or bus – despite its inconvenience (and despite being aware of studies that show air travel is far safer).

Various forms of therapy can help. One of the most effective is called desensitization or exposure therapy, where the person is *gradually* exposed to the feared stimulus, while at the same time discussing their fears with a therapist. In other words, the person with a snake phobia might begin by looking at pictures of snakes until she feels comfortable with that stage. The next step might be to see one in a terrarium, and perhaps ultimately work up to handling one. By slowly introducing the stimulus in less intense situations – and by exploring what specifically prompts the anxiety – many people can overcome their fears.

Obsessive-compulsive Disorder

When the film *As Good As It Gets* was released, much was written about Jack Nicholson's portrayal of an author with obsessive-compulsive disorder. Nicholson repeatedly engaged in elaborate rituals that would appear nonsensical to an observer, but which held a great deal of meaning for his character. Things like avoiding cracks on the sidewalk, locking his apartment door in an unusual fashion – even the way he arranged his cutlery. He was obsessive about it, and felt compelled to complete the rituals.

For 2% of the people watching the film, Nicholson's actions held a personal resonance. Because that's the percentage of people, at least according to a major Australian study, thought to have the disorder.

Most of us have rituals – odd little things we may do in the hope they will bring us good luck, or help avoid bad luck. A person with obsessive-compulsive disorder might be thought of as someone who does this to the extreme, and with the *knowledge* that the rituals have no effect on reality.

Diagnostic manuals, in an effort to draw the line between simple quirks and disorder, point out that someone with obsessive-compulsive disorder is powerless to stop their actions, and that those actions consume at least an hour of time in a given day. (The choice of "one hour" as a defining characteristic is another good example of how diagnostic criteria can sometimes appear arbitrary.)

Nonetheless, there are cases where these rituals can grossly interfere with living. We learned of a successful Canadian businesswoman who started getting up earlier every day to apply her makeup. As the disorder progressed, she was spending hours in front of her bathroom mirror – starting in the middle of the night. She knew it was irrational, but felt powerless to stop it.

Psychotherapy has been shown to be quite effective in treating the *compulsion* half of the equation, and antidepressants often help reduce the *obsessive* patterns of thinking. For this reason, many use a combination of both.

Posttraumatic Stress Disorder (PTSD)

World War II has been described as a seminal event – not only in global history, but also in psychiatry. Countless soldiers were stricken with invisible injuries, psychic wounds that resisted healing.

Although shell shock had been observed in World War I, the amount of psychological damage inflicted in World War II prompted some in psychiatry to reassess their traditional views. Many had previously tended to put people into one of two categories: mentally well and mentally ill. Yet here was evidence, *en masse*, that circumstances – environment – could drive someone from a state of sound mental health to a state of astonishing disability. This led to the theory that mental health and mental ill-health could be viewed as a single continuum – with no demarcation line.

Fast forward to Vietnam. Once again, we saw people return from a faraway place, forever altered. And yet there was no medical name we could affix to the debilitating symptoms that plagued veterans: the waking nightmares, the flashbacks, the jumbled nerves – symptoms that left many unable to function as they had before.

Veterans felt this condition needed recognition. These weren't "weak" people who had been affected – and their symptoms didn't fade with the passage of time. The lack of a diagnostic category not only meant problems collecting disability benefits, it also meant no one would be carefully researching the phenomenon and looking for effective methods of treatment. "Treatment," for many vets, meant escaping into the numbing depths of a bottle. And so they lobbied – effectively – for their symptoms to be acknowledged.

Thus was born posttraumatic stress disorder (PTSD).

One of the more notable cases in Canada is that of retired lieutenant-general Roméo Dallaire, who led a UN mission to Rwanda in 1994. Dallaire, quite simply, saw too much. Since then he's been diagnosed with the disorder and has spoken publicly about its personal impact. He's experienced waking nightmares, has had commonplace sights or smells in Canada transport him back to the hell he witnessed. Following testimony at a UN war-crimes tribunal in 1998, Dallaire told a Canadian Press reporter, "At one point yesterday, I had the sense of smell of the slaughter – I don't know how. What we saw was beyond belief."

Dallaire clearly went through hell. But you don't have to be a soldier to experience these symptoms – or to receive a diagnosis. Many Canadians witness or endure traumatic events that change us profoundly. In fact, some of the newest Canadians – refugees from strife-torn or oppressive nations – are displaying symptoms of this disorder. Mental health workers from Vancouver, Calgary, and Toronto have all told the authors of this phenomenon. One doctor, who works on a psychiatric ward in a general hospital, says, "It's become a United Nations in here."

People who work in the emergency services are also prone to this disorder. Police officers, firefighters, and paramedics routinely find that, following a particularly difficult call, the event comes back to haunt them. Almost literally. Victims of violent crime or abuse can also suffer the following symptoms of PTSD.

- You can't get the experience out of your head. Distressing thoughts, images, or recollections seem to keep intruding on your thoughts no matter what you do to keep them at bay.
- You're plagued by recurring dreams or nightmares of the event. They may awaken you in a startled state.
- Small noises might spook you or make you jump – responses markedly more exaggerated than they would have been prior to the event.
- You may experience flashbacks of the event or have a sense of reliving the traumatic experience.
- These symptoms last more than one month (three months is considered chronic).

Many believe the most effective treatment is to talk out your feelings about the experience. There's evidence that the sooner a person is able to "unload" following the incident, the better the outcome. New Brunswick has an innovative program, Critical Incident Stress Management, geared toward the general public. Police and other emergency personnel in the province distribute cards with a 1-800 number to people who've witnessed or endured traumatic events.

In February 2000, the Canadian federal government recognized PTSD as a disability, extending benefits to several thousand peacekeepers and Gulf War veterans.

SUBSTANCE ABUSE

Traditionally, we've tended to erect artificial fences between the worlds of addiction and mental health. Many Canadian services, including community agencies, reflect this perceived division, sending people to one set of professionals to treat their addiction, another to address their mental health.

Now, however, there's a growing emphasis on dealing with both issues at once, a concept known as "integrated treatment."

Substance abuse and mental disorders are usually flip sides of the same coin; the two, if both present in the same person, are largely inextricable. People with depression, for example, often turn to alcohol as a way of temporarily easing their pain. Conversely, many people who drink too much become depressed because of the effects of the alcohol.

Substance abuse – particularly alcohol – is also a factor in numerous suicides. Many people are severely impaired at the moment they end their lives. Chronic use of alcohol or other substances can also lead to symptoms that mimic other psychiatric disorders – a diagnostician's nightmare if he or she is unaware of the abuse problem. And while it's generally agreed that moderate alcohol consumption is not harmful, consuming more than fourteen drinks per week is often regarded as an indicator of a potential problem.

In the diagnostic world, however, there's no such marker. The following criteria for abuse apply whether it's fine Scotch, crack cocaine, or airplane glue. And you only have to exhibit one symptom to qualify.

- Your recurrent use of the substance is really interfering with your life – on the job, at home, at school. You might be missing work because of your substance abuse, or your performance at work is substandard. At home, you could be neglecting your kids, your household, your spouse. You might be spending money on the substance that should be earmarked for other priorities.
- You use the substance, repeatedly, in situations where its use could lead to physical injury: you drive while impaired, operate heavy machinery, stagger around in traffic, and so on. (One study of private plane crashes in the United States found that alcohol was a factor in 10% of accidents.) Alternatively, you continue to use the substance despite knowing it may be detrimental to an existing psychological or physical condition (such as alcohol use with hepatitis C).
- Your repeated use of the substance has led to legal or disciplinary problems, such as an arrest.

- You continue to use the substance despite repeated social or interpersonal problems resulting from its use. For example, you have recurrent arguments, perhaps even physical fights, with a spouse over substance abuse (or while impaired), yet you *continue* to use the substance regardless of those consequences.

Medical treatment for substance abuse frequently consists of intense psychotherapy, often in group settings. In cases where the person shows signs of physical addiction, medication is often used for a brief period to ease the symptoms of withdrawal before starting therapy.

While most Canadian communities have addiction programs funded by provincial health departments, don't forget about the important role self-help can play. Groups such as Alcoholics Anonymous (AA) and its spinoffs, which offer peer support within a non-denominational spiritual framework, have been tremendously successful around the world. Numbers for AA can be found in your local phone book.

EATING DISORDERS

"You can never be too rich or too thin."
    – Wallis Simpson, the Duchess of Windsor

There's been much in the media in recent years about eating disorders. Whether it's Anne Murray and her daughter going public over the teen's struggle with anorexia, or speculation over the thin frame of TV star Calista Flockhart (*Ally McBeal*), these disorders have become mainstream news.

The coverage may give the impression anorexia and bulimia are very common, but the jury is out on precisely *how* common. Some studies have indicated rates as low as one person with anorexia in every hundred thousand – though more recent work in Western countries has produced rates of between 1 and 2%. Bulimia is far more prevalent;

one Australian study found that a staggering one in six female high school students reported having experienced symptoms.

Not surprisingly, prevalence appears to be higher in fashion-conscious, advertising-saturated nations like our own. Thin, to our Western eyes, often means beautiful.

These are not disorders to take lightly. Mortality rates for those with anorexia range from 5% to as high as 18%.

Anorexia nervosa is a ceaseless pursuit of thinness. Body image can become so distorted that the individual, despite being drastically underweight, is convinced they need to lose more weight. It is most common among teenaged females, though up to 10% of cases are males.

People suffering from anorexia, unlike someone suffering from starvation, tend to be energetic, often hyperactive. It's often observed that their eyes seem quite "bright." They do not show the usual apathy and fatigue found in someone who is starving. They may, in addition to severely limiting food intake (and obsessively watching calories), strenuously exercise to lose additional weight. Typically, those with the disorder are at least 15% underweight for their age and height; they often refuse any attempt to encourage them to put on pounds. In fact, they frequently display an intense *fear* of gaining weight or becoming obese.

As the disorder progresses, most young women develop amenorrhea – they cease to menstruate. Malnutrition can lead to kidney dysfunction, urinary tract infections, and colon damage – along with seizures, muscle spasms, or cramps. Concentration and rational thinking can also be impaired, simply because there aren't enough nutrients to feed the brain.

Bulimia, which is marked by binge eating and purging, often coexists with anorexia, though people with bulimia are not necessarily anorexic (and vice versa). Those diagnosed with the disorder typically follow a pattern: at least twice a week, over a period lasting at least three months, they gorge, eating far more at a single sitting than other people would under normal circumstances. Many report that they "can't control" this eating behaviour, that it feels like they're somehow being compelled to eat unusual amounts. They also try to compensate for the binge by taking measures to ensure it won't result in weight gain. They may induce vomiting, take laxatives or diuretics, or exercise to an extreme. As with anorexia, there is a distortion of self-image.

Bulimia causes many of the same physical problems as anorexia. In addition, frequent vomiting in severe bulimia is likely to erode dental enamel. Many a parent first picked up on the problem by questioning their child about teeth that started to turn grey. The disorder can also cause swelling of the salivary glands, and a chronic sore throat. In serious cases, the stomach can rupture.

Quite often, depression, anxiety, or substance dependence accompanies these disorders. Precisely what *causes* them in the first place is uncertain, though many people with anorexia lack a sense of control in their lives. Food intake is the one thing they *can* control. Other common themes include poor communication within the family or a recent significant loss.

Psychotherapy is considered a critical part of treatment, though individuals with co-existing depression or anxiety often respond to medication. Group therapy, in which those with the disorder and their peers can talk in a safe and trusting environment, is frequently used and can produce positive results. Family counselling is often an integral part of the treatment plan.

People in a state of severe malnourishment, however, gain little benefit from psychotherapy until the body has a sufficient level of nutrients. Those seriously underweight often require hospitalization until they've returned to a level where their health is not jeopardized. In life-threatening situations, nutrients sometimes have to be pumped into the person through a nasal gastric tube.

PERSONALITY DISORDERS

As the name suggests, these are disorders of personality. In the very broadest sense, they refer to people who just don't seem to "fit in" with life. So great is the mismatch between their behaviour and the culturally accepted norms or expectations that such people, and often those around them, suffer significant distress as a result.

All of us have personality traits. These are, by the time we reach adulthood, pretty much ingrained ways in which we experience, react to, and interact with the various people and events that life throws at us. Such traits comprise much of our world view. They define *who we are*. Those with a personality disorder don't view or react to the world in a "normal" way. They could be thought of as people whose traits are so rigid – whose mismatch is so great – that their lives are impaired.

It's a quirky one, this. The DSM lists ten different personality disorders, each with its own title and diagnostic criteria. Those diagnoses tend to hinge on the *nature* of the mismatch, so it's worth emphasizing, with this category in particular, that the titles used are descriptive, often disputed, labels. For example, a person who feels so inadequate or fearful of rejection that they shun many social situations could be diagnosed with avoidant personality disorder. A layperson might describe that same person, perhaps with equal validity, as "painfully shy."

Borderline Personality Disorder

A very controversial and common diagnosis within this category is borderline personality disorder – controversial because many people who have experienced sexual or physical abuse exhibit one of its defining symptoms, self-harm behaviour. This is the cutting or mutilation of oneself as an expression of anger, a cry for help, the physical manifestation of immense emotional pain. The controversy arises because what the manuals might call a "disorder" would be labelled by many others, particularly those who work with victims of abuse, as legitimate pain or grief.

Roughly 75% of all those who receive the diagnosis are women.

People with this label frequently have volatile mood swings, persistent difficulties with interpersonal relationships, and an unstable sense of who they are. They're often frantic in their efforts to prevent abandonment in a relationship, whether that abandonment is real or imagined. An example might be the woman (or man) who becomes frenzied when their partner can't be reached by phone. Most of us would simply call later; a person with borderline personality disorder might leave fifteen panicked messages, travel across town to see if they can locate their partner, or maybe hurl the phone across the room in a disproportionate burst of anger.

Clinicians will want to make sure that such symptoms aren't better accounted for by other disorders, such as a major depression or substance abuse. There is thought to be significant misdiagnosis because of failure to recognize other underlying disorders. Up to 10% of people with this diagnosis complete suicide.

To receive a diagnosis of borderline personality disorder, you'll have to satisfy five of the following criteria.

- You have a pattern of suicidal behaviour, which could include making threats of suicide or repeatedly harming or mutilating yourself.
- Your personal relationships tend to be both intense and unstable. You alternate, sometimes frequently, between thinking you're with the perfect partner and thinking you can't stand them.
- You'll go to extremes to avoid being abandoned. This potential abandonment can be either real, or – as the phone example illustrates – imagined.
- You feel "empty" for extended periods much of the time.
- You've got an explosive temper that you can't seem to control. Little things can cause you to explode in a rage or even engage in physical fighting.

- Your mood is frequently unstable for brief and intense periods. You may feel overwhelmingly anxious, sad, or irritable – feelings that can last anywhere from a few hours to a few days.
- You don't have a good sense of who you are. Your self-image is unstable and can change rapidly.
- You can be very impulsive in ways that are damaging to yourself. For example, you might go on an eating or drinking binge, drive your car recklessly, decide to have sexual relations with a stranger.

Again, this disorder is a very controversial one. Pat Fisher, a clinical psychologist in Vancouver, agrees that the diagnosis is "hugely overused." She believes most – but not all – people given this label have been incorrectly diagnosed. Yet she also thinks the label has merit.

"There is a group of people, a much smaller group of people, who really classically fulfil the borderline personality disorder category."

As with many psychiatric disorders, there are a couple of schools of thought regarding appropriate treatment. Some practitioners believe medication has a primary role to play, while others focus on psychotherapy. Some research shows that the best results are achieved when both are used in combination. The actual medication prescribed can vary from case to case, depending on symptoms, ranging all the way from anti-depressants through to low doses of antipsychotics. Some physicians, however, warn against treatment consisting solely of drugs. Psychosocial intervention is generally considered a crucial part of helping someone with this diagnosis.

It's worth noting that people who truly fulfil the criteria of borderline personality disorder often have rocky relationships with their psychiatrists or psychologists. The intense and unstable bonds they form with people outside of therapy can also occur during sessions. Often, they develop what has been described as a love-hate relationship with caregivers. When things go well, the physician or psychologist is a hero or rescuer. When things go poorly, they are often blamed. (Many people with this diagnosis simply cannot or will not participate in long-term therapy.)

As for the specific type of psychotherapy, that, too, can vary according to symptoms, the practitioner, and the individual's preference. Cognitive-behavioural therapy, which attempts to short-circuit negative thinking patterns, has been found to be quite useful with this diagnosis, but is by no means the sole option. There is frequently an emphasis on reality-oriented problem solving – helping the person learn to deal with issues in their lives before they become overwhelming.

Antisocial Personality Disorder

In the public eye, this is a label that stands out. It refers to people sometimes called "sociopaths."

These are, in a word, people who don't subscribe to the same moral code as the rest of us. An estimated 75% of the prison population in the United States would satisfy the criteria for this disorder – and it's easy to see why. They're basically people who, since the age of fifteen, have had a habit of getting into trouble, over and over again.

Most with this diagnosis come from severely disturbed home settings, and it's not uncommon for one or both parents to display the same symptoms. Alcohol and drug abuse frequently coexist, and can worsen antisocial behaviour. To get this diagnosis, you'd have to be at least eighteen years old and satisfy at least three of the following criteria.

- You repeatedly do things that get you arrested. Even after being arrested or punished, you continue to break the law.
- You lie and it doesn't bother you. You don't mind conning people.
- You're impulsive and can't plan ahead.
- You're aggressive, irritable, pugnacious. The kind of guy (or gal) who gets into bar fights at the drop of a hat.

- You show no regard for the welfare of others. In fact, you do things that show a wanton disregard for the safety of other people.
- You've got a pattern of being irresponsible. You can't hold a steady job or meet financial obligations.
- You feel no remorse over what you've done; you don't care who gets hurt or how much pain you cause. Your conscience, in this respect, is absent. (Some people with this diagnosis do report feelings of guilt. However, their guilt does not cause them to change their behaviour.)
- Your actions didn't occur during a psychosis. You knew what you were doing – and did it anyway.

Although much of the evidence indicates these characteristics are the direct result of environment, several twin studies suggest there may be other factors at play. Identical twins (who are genetically the same) are more likely to share the disorder than fraternal twins. Some longer-term studies have also shown that children of criminals, when adopted early in life by non-relatives, are more likely to become criminals than are adopted children whose biological parents were law-abiding.

All personality disorders tend to be somewhat difficult to treat, because you're dealing with the oft-inflexible way someone *is*, rather than an intrusion of mood or anxiety. Some therapies focus on techniques to alter behaviour (like anger management) – while others try to explore deeper issues thought to have helped form the personality. Symptoms of antisocial personality disorder tend to fade as the person ages, and it's hypothesized these traits simply "burn out" in some people.

SCHIZOPHRENIA

This is, bar none, the most serious disorder in the mental health world. Its symptoms can be bizarre and frightening, both to the sufferer and those close to them. It is often referred to as "youth's greatest disabler," because it commonly strikes in the late teens and early twenties. As with other mental disorders, there is currently no "cure" – although between one-quarter and one-third of people with the diagnosis find their symptoms disappear over time. It is quite possible, but not yet proven, that this group of people is suffering from a different disorder. The authors have met several consumers who displayed temporary schizophrenia-like symptoms during a difficult period in their lives.

Not so long ago, parents were directly blamed for their child's schizophrenia. There was, as late as the 1970s, an accepted theory that personality flaws of the mother – the so-called "schizophrenogenic mother" – were the real cause. One woman, now a prominent mental health activist, recalls the words of the doctor when her son was diagnosed: " 'No wonder with a mother like you.' I went home and cried for five years. Then I got very, very angry."

Parents' groups, understandably, have been distancing themselves from the notion that they are in any way responsible for their loved-one's disorder. The U.S.-based National Alliance for the Mentally Ill (NAMI) now refers to schizophrenia and bipolar disorder as NBD – neurobiological disorders. The Schizophrenia Society of Canada frequently refers to it as a "biochemical brain disease." But there is still no conclusive evidence on precisely what causes this mystifying disorder.

The course of schizophrenia can vary tremendously. It can build slowly over a long period – "gradual onset" – or appear very quickly. Many people respond well to antipsychotic medication; others suffer severe and repeated psychotic episodes that are resistant to drugs. There are even individuals who find their symptoms manageable – voices and all – without the use of medication. Are these people all suffering from precisely the same disorder? It's not known for sure, but many leading researchers now believe that what we call schizophrenia is actually several distinct disorders. One form, for example, may be related to a virus or infection in utero, passed on while a fetus is still in the womb, but does not trigger disorder until adolescence or later.

Within the broad range of schizophrenia-related disorders, there are two clinical terms that often create confusion: positive symptoms and negative symptoms. "Positive" does not mean good; it means symptoms that are present but should not be there, like delusions, hallucinations, and thought disorders. "Negative" refers to the *absence* of behaviour that *should* be there. These include a dulling or flattening of emotions or emotional expression, an overall lack of motivation, and apathy; the absence of normal drives, interests, and expression (providing these negative symptoms have not been caused by medication or other substances).

The many symptoms associated with schizophrenia are listed fully in diagnostic manuals. What we'll describe here commonly occurs in what might be called classic schizophrenia.

- Delusions: You cling to unusual beliefs despite all evidence to the contrary. A licence-plate number, for example, may be interpreted as a signal from space aliens. People with the disorder frequently suffer from delusions involving persecution, where they may believe they're being spied on, plotted against, or having their thoughts controlled by others.
- Hallucinations: Most commonly, this means hearing voices. The voices may seem to be coming from inside your head – or from elsewhere. On occasion, you may hear two or more voices in conversation with one another. These auditory hallucinations frequently involve hearing "messages" being broadcast from the radio or television. Sometimes voices can be comforting or reassuring; sometimes they can be extremely threatening and frightening. One Calgary man who showed up at an emergency ward had for months been hearing an insistent voice commanding, "Kill yourself." Some people with the disorder have a broad range of visual hallucinations, which can be disturbingly real. The disorder can also involve tactile sensations; it might feel like your skin is covered with insects, or there's some foreign presence inside your body.

- Disorder of thoughts/speech: Your thinking process can be extremely fragmented. You may speak in ways where nothing seems logically connected; the link is often so tangential that it's impossible for other people to understand what you're talking about. You may also frequently respond to things in an emotionally inappropriate way. For example, during a discussion of a tragic topic you might burst into laughter.
- Negative symptoms: As discussed above, you may feel apathetic, experience a dulling of overall emotional response.

If, in addition to these symptoms, you experience mania, depression, or a mixture of both, you may receive a diagnosis of schizoaffective disorder.

Because of the often insidious nature of schizophrenia – the fact that the symptoms can creep along rather subtly over a long time – many people are not diagnosed until they are in an acute phase. Conversely, because some of the symptoms can occur in other disorders involving psychosis, people may be incorrectly diagnosed.

Health Canada, in co-operation with the Schizophrenia Society of Canada, publishes *Schizophrenia: A Handbook for Families*. This manual contains a useful list of early warning signs that family members felt, in retrospect, were the first indication of the disorder. Available through Health Canada, your local chapter of the Schizophrenia Society, and online, the book also contains useful tips for coping and for defusing crises. It reflects the collective wisdom of many Canadian families who have dealt with the disorder – though it contains far less from the perspective of the person diagnosed.

Common treatment for schizophrenia involves the use of antipsychotic medications, sometimes known as "neuroleptics." Though often effective, these powerful drugs can have potent side effects. Recent advances have reduced many adverse effects, and many people report that they can work and function well on low doses. Indeed, many in the medical community now recognize that people have historically received higher doses of these medications than was necessary to control psychotic symptoms. Certain forms of psychotherapy are often recommended as an adjunct treatment. We'll cover more ground on medications in Chapter 8, but there's one more thing worth mentioning.

Many people, invariably those who do not have the diagnosis, take the view that "as long as they take their drugs, things will be fine." Medication, if we adhere to the biopsychosocial model, addresses just one component. When society, as it does, continues to marginalize, underhouse, and underemploy those diagnosed with this disorder, we can not possibly expect them to become truly "well."

Nor should the responsibility of a caring physician be limited to a prescription pad. Dr. Mary Seeman, a well-known authority on schizophrenia, concurs.

"I know that if I just give them drugs and don't give them something else – a feeling of safety, of hope, of security – if I don't give them all of that and see them through it and share their burden," she says, "then the drug alone isn't going to do anything."

A CAUTIONARY TALE

With any of the disorders discussed above, we must be careful not to assume we've got all the answers. While the authors don't dispute the existence of mental disorders, we've certainly met people who do. The survivor movement cites personal experiences of the medical profession's rush to diagnose and medicate. This seems to be particularly true with schizophrenia: any time someone says they hear voices, it's often assumed that's the diagnosis.

We believe there may be other reasons why some people hear voices – ranging from extreme trauma to heartbreaking loneliness. A symptom-based approach rarely acknowledges the full range of human experience, in all its complexity and diversity. The example of a native Canadian woman springs to mind.

She was being held, involuntarily, at a psychiatric hospital because she was hearing voices. All of the clinical symptoms indicated schizophrenia, and hospital staff were adamant she required medical treatment and continued hospitalization. The woman, however, viewed these voices from a spiritual perspective and wanted to seek the advice of a traditional native healer.

Dr. Ed Connors, a psychologist of aboriginal descent, was involved with the case. "There wasn't a lot of change in her condition while in the institution," he says. When eventually released, however, she sought the help of a traditional healer, who interpreted the voices from a spiritual perspective. Dr. Connors ran into her years later; she was symptom-free.

"None of what she had been presenting before was there," says Dr. Connors. "The elder . . . understood it in relation to spirits that she was carrying that she needed to free herself from.

"In her estimation," continues Dr. Connors, the traditional healing was "what really made the changes for her and allowed her to find what we would refer to as sanity. She was healed, cured, through the treatment."

Dr. Connors cautions that medication is usually a critical component of treatment for this disorder. In this case, however, it was not.

The story serves to remind us of an important truth: Mental disorder is often highly individual.

S H E R Y L ' S   S T O R Y

I have been diagnosed by three different psychiatrists over a period of fifteen years as a person who suffers from chronic low-grade depression and obsessive-compulsive disorder (OCD).

What finally brought my condition to the forefront was the onset of OCD at age seventeen (I am now thirty-two). The episode was so severe I was completely incapacitated. The obsessions were overwhelming and terrifying. I had no idea what was happening. My mother, a devout Catholic, kept screaming at me to "give your head a shake and snap out of it." I did not know at the time that my father was under treatment for depression and OCD. The worst part is that no one spoke about it. To this day, my mother does not know why my father was in therapy, and she thinks that his compulsive behaviour is "funny."

The first episode prompted a visit to my father's doctor. He was the first to diagnose me. He prescribed Anafranil for the obsessions. I found it difficult to deal with the side effects of the drug, and after a few weeks decided to work at managing the obsessions without drugs. I read everything I could on the disease and worked hard using behaviour-modification techniques (I devised my own). I was determined that I could not, would not, let this thing beat me. This particular episode lasted nearly one year. Recovery from it was roughly three years. I found my university studies particularly helpful, as the intense studying refocused my mind. I thought I was "cured."

At the age of twenty-seven, during the first year of my marriage, it happened again. My husband did not believe in the existence of mental illness and thought it was a sign of "character weakness." Yes, my very own husband. As a result of his feelings and my desire to prove myself worthy in his eyes, my illness went untreated. My family physician was urging me to take Paxil and to see someone. I told him, "My husband won't allow it."

Over the next two years, I lived in a vacuum, hiding my illness. I felt so alone. At this time I was obsessing about suffocating and developing breast tumours. I was in and out of doctors' offices and hospital for tests. (At the beginning of an episode you don't know if it's the disease or not; you truly believe that these things are happening to you. Soon it becomes so ridiculous that you realize it is the disease.) Fortunately, I had one caring physician who was patient enough to coach me through my hysteria.

Dealing with the obsession of developing breast lumps was a nightmare. Imagine walking into my office to find me constantly performing a self-exam. My mind kept telling me to "Check again because you missed it. It's there, oh another is forming. Feel it, it's there." Over and over again. My breasts were so swollen. I couldn't let my husband touch me for fear that a lump would start to grow.

I was working as a director of planning and investments at a communications firm (I am a professional accountant) when I knew it was time to get help. I was sitting in my office and I felt the walls closing in on me. I was starting to believe I was hearing voices, on top of the obsessions that were consuming my life. I became so afraid for myself and my life that I went to see my doctor.

That summer I began taking Paxil. I am still on it, and can say that I have had no OCD symptoms for three years. The Paxil also manages the low-grade depression.

My husband was enraged by the medication. In his eyes, I was defective. The wedge between us was undeniable. Here I was, fighting for my sanity, and the man I loved believed his wife was defective.

I refused to stop taking the medication, as it was helping. He, too, conceded I was doing much better. But he wanted me to stop taking it – thought I was "cured."

I won't stop taking it, as I cannot imagine ever having to go through another episode.

My husband has since left me. I have discovered that OCD was present on my father's side for at least three generations.

Recently, I was attending a company function with my boss here in Vancouver. He teased me about the way I eat. He was chuckling to another fellow and said to me, "You know, you remind me of that movie with Jack Nicholson, As Good As It Gets. You know, the guy that suffered from that disease . . ."

I said, "Oh, you mean obsessive-compulsive disorder?" To myself I laughed, You guys have no idea!

Today, I am healthy. I still have days where I look at my pill bottle and think, Do I still need these? I'm fine. Then I remember how sick I could get again, and quite frankly, life is too short to give another two or three years away to an OCD episode.

CHAPTER SIX

Getting Help

Break your leg, develop a hacking cough or rash, and you know what to do. You see your family doctor, who fixes the problem or refers you to a specialist who can. Easy, right?

Unfortunately, in the world of *mental* health, the path to treatment is rarely so straightforward. Help is out there, but finding it – finding the services that are right for *you* – is a bit like navigating a maze. How do you go about locating a good doctor? What is "self-help"? Is hospital the only option in a crisis? Is there anyone out there who truly understands what you're going through?

This chapter will help you navigate the maze. We won't recommend any one treatment for any one disorder – those are choices only you can make. But we can let you know what's out there, including mental health agencies and support groups. Each step of the way, we'll tell you what should happen – and some of the ways in which things can go wrong. And we hope we'll provide some encouragement to keep you on the path. Because seeking help – of whatever kind – is the first step toward wellness.

PARALLEL WORLDS

What's called the mental health "system" actually consists of two worlds. One is the world many of us have heard of – physicians, psychiatrists, psychologists, and hospitals. This is the "formal" system. It's a critical component of care, and the place to go for medication, psychotherapy, and many other mainstream treatment options.

But there's another, "informal" system out there, which offers different kinds of support. This is the world where you'll find the warm embrace of peers and the collective wisdom of consumers and family members who've gone before you. It's the place where consumer advocacy takes shape. And it's where you'll realize that not only are you not alone, you're actually part of a very big and welcoming crowd.

In this chapter, we'll describe the basics of both of these worlds. But it's worth noting that while these systems are complementary, there's often a communications breakdown between the two. Your physician may be unaware that a terrific self-help group exists mere blocks from your home. Your psychiatrist may not know that your local Canadian Mental Health Association (CMHA) branch is offering a workshop on job skills. Likewise, your local self-help group might not have heard about the latest day-treatment program for depression being offered by the hospital. In other words, you'll have to do some legwork to learn what's available near you.

Informed consumers find the best of *both* worlds, taking advantage of the mix of supports that suit them best. Supports like the mobile crisis teams that serve much of rural Manitoba, helping people in their own homes. The more than five hundred self-help groups in Nova Scotia, some 20% of which are devoted *solely* to mental health. The many drop-ins across the country that offer everything from a coffee and chat through to organized government lobbying. . . . These are options that reflect the many ways of looking at – and approaching – mental disorders.

Getting help shouldn't just be about some professional telling you what to do. *You* should be the primary player, the person who comes to understand the reasons behind what ails you, and the routes to overcoming it. What feels right for one person will be completely inappropriate to another. So trust yourself – it's your recovery.

Before we start exploring some of these options – both from the formal and informal systems – it's worth emphasizing a few points.

- Become an informed consumer. At every stage in your treatment, it's crucial that you know as much as you possibly can about mental disorder. Read widely on the subject, search the Internet, visit local support groups (many of which have reading rooms), and talk to fellow consumers.
- Reach out to people you trust. Confide in close friends and family members who can listen with respect, and offer comfort. Loved ones know you in ways that no professional can. For this reason alone, they are perhaps the most crucial sources of support.
- Be patient. And, if necessary, *push* for the services you need. When it comes to getting help, it's up to you – and the people closest to you – to expect the best and ensure you receive just that.

WHO GETS CARE?

Research suggests that the earlier a person gets treatment, the better the prognosis will be. Remission of symptoms is faster, and relapses are fewer. This sounds like common sense, but it has only recently become a priority among mental health professionals. The buzzword now is "early intervention" – assessing, treating, and supporting consumers as soon as signs of disorder show up.

The truth is, we still have a long way to go. People take a long time before they look for help. The CMHA's Early Intervention Study interviewed 115 consumers and family members in British Columbia about their experiences with the mental health system. It found that, on average, from the first onset of disorder, it took people with schizophrenia three years to access treatment. For people with mood disorders, it took seven to eight years.

Worse still, many people seek no help at all. Studies suggest that, on average, only one-quarter of Canadians with a mental disorder reach out. Bill Ashdown, president of the Mood Disorders Association of Canada, estimates that only one-third of people with depression seek help.

"The other two out of three, particularly if they're men, tend to suffer in silence. And they tend to self-treat using other means. And obviously the most popular means in the adult male population, unfortunately, is alcohol."

What makes these statistics so tragic is that mental disorder is very treatable. The vast majority of people, when they finally do get help, respond well and recover.

So why does it take so long to get there? The B.C. Early Intervention Study identified three crucial areas, each of which we'll discuss in turn.

Recognizing the Problem

As our own story shows, it can take some time to figure out what's going on. Family members may notice something's wrong, but then minimize or misinterpret the symptoms. He's on drugs, they think. She's going through a phase. Acting up, being difficult.

"I thought he might be sick," one family member told the B.C. study. "But his grandparents thought he was lazy and taking advantage."

Through lack of knowledge or experience, this may be all that comes to mind. Maybe, too, there's an element of denial; nobody wants to think their loved one could be seriously ill. Either way, mental disorder is so seldom discussed and so widely misunderstood that when it does strike, people rarely have the information they need to recognize it.

So-called "gatekeepers" – family doctors, teachers, or counsellors – can also misinterpret the symptoms, or fail to notice them. In school, a student might be expelled for bad behaviour instead of being given support. At the doctor's office, a depressed person complaining of headaches might be given an MRI scan, which reveals nothing wrong.

Consumers may notice changes in themselves – shifts in mood or thought or behaviour. But often they are unable to make sense of those changes.

"I knew there was something wrong, but I couldn't put my finger on it," one consumer told the B.C. study.

"I thought they [the voices] would go away, so I kept on working," said another.

So how do you make sense of what's happening to you? When is the problem bad enough to seek help? Symptoms will vary with each disorder, and it's important not to try to diagnose yourself. What you *can* decide is whether the problem – regardless of what it is – significantly interferes with your life. This is the *key* question to ask yourself. Are your thoughts so dark that your work or family life is suffering? Is the anxiety so troubling that you never get a good night's sleep?

Of equal importance is duration. Have these feelings or symptoms lasted weeks? Months? Have people close to you expressed concern or worry over your well-being? If the answer is yes, the problem may well have exceeded your ability to cope.

Ultimately, the decision is yours and yours alone – but here's a general rule of thumb:

> *If your thoughts, feelings, or behaviours are significantly impairing your life . . . it may be time to seek help*

Building Motivation

Even if you feel you *do* need help, you may be reluctant to ask for it. Here's where public attitudes and misconceptions come into play. Who wants to admit to a mental health problem in a world where the mentally disordered are feared, despised, and shunned? Who dares admit to being crazy, nuts, or loony?

"Quite often it requires a real act of will for somebody to reach out and get help," says Bill Ashdown, "because essentially it's going against everything that they've learned, growing up."

Some people choose the fix-themselves approach. Not wanting to be judged or show their weakness, they try anything and everything on their own. Going to the doctor becomes the absolute last straw.

"What you see, in general," says Dr. Nady el-Guebaly, past president of the Canadian Psychiatric Association (CPA), "is people who have tried a number of things: take a rest, take a vacation, try and change this, get a hobby . . . and then they go to their physician and say, 'By the way, I have tried a, b, c, and d, and it looks like it's not happening.'"

Other people try to tough it out. They may think they deserve their misery, that they're bad or weak people, that nothing can help them anyway. Depressed or anxious or fearful, they struggle along for weeks or months or years, failing to realize there are solutions.

"I thought it was just me, just the way I was," one consumer told us.

Too often, what finally leads to treatment is a drastic worsening of symptoms (for example, psychosis or a suicide attempt) or of situation (losing a job or a relationship). People wind up in hospital, severely unwell. In the CMHA B.C. study, 60% of participants' first contact with the system was a hospital emergency ward.

That's why it's important to get help *before* things get that bad. Many consumers and family members recognize, in retrospect, that there were warning signs early on, and wish they'd acted sooner. That includes the authors of this book!

Don't allow symptoms to drastically worsen before seeking help

Accessing Care
This is, without a doubt, the greatest frustration consumers voiced to us. Accessing not just any old care but the kind of care that works – that makes *you* feel better – can be extremely

trying. People tell us that the system treats them as illnesses, not as individuals – that it fails to recognize their unique and distinct needs.

"The system is just not set up to meet people on their terms," says Eric Macnaughton, author of the B.C. Early Intervention Study. "It's so difficult to navigate through, to find just where to look for help."

We say this not to discourage you, but rather to prepare you for the task ahead. And to encourage you to keep trying.

THE "FORMAL" SYSTEM

Family Doctors

Not everyone tries this route first. Some people prefer to speak first with a trusted minister, rabbi, or other spiritual adviser. Many of them are trained counsellors who can discuss treatment options with you and even provide referrals.

Still, the family doctor is probably the most common first point of contact with the health-care system, if only because almost all Canadians have one.

General practitioners (GPs) deal with mental health issues so frequently, you needn't feel embarrassed or ashamed to describe your symptoms. In one Ontario survey, family doctors reported spending up to half of their time "identifying and helping their patients deal with mental illnesses."

Ideally, your family doctor will have a complete record of your medical history. He or she should give you a full examination to rule out any physical ailments that might be the root of your troubles. Depression, for example, can be triggered by a thyroid problem. Even if you don't have overt full symptoms, a check-up is still a good idea. This often includes blood work and neurological testing.

Once the doctor has ruled out any physical troubles, mental disorder becomes a more likely explanation. Your family doctor should conduct a detailed interview – about your symptoms and the life circumstances surrounding them – before reaching a diagnosis. Then there should be a discussion about the reasons for reaching that diagnosis, and about the range of treatment options available. It may take several visits before all this has been accomplished.

If you're content with the explanations you've been given, and with the course of treatment you embark on, this may be all the professional help you need. Your doctor will arrange for follow-up visits to track your recovery. Many people with depression, for example, rely solely on their GP – and a growing number of GPs offer psychotherapy as well.

Some consumers tell us they were more than satisfied with their family doctor's knowledge, dedication, and care. It's worth noting, though, that not everyone feels that way. Levels of knowledge and understanding vary widely among GPs. In medical school, training focuses more on physical than on mental health. Consumers frequently report that their problems were either dismissed or misdiagnosed, particularly where symptoms were atypical.

"I worked at a TV and radio station, and I thought they were transmitting my thoughts over the air," one person told the B.C. Early Intervention Study. "I went to my doctor . . . and he said the problem was because my husband was very assertive and I needed help getting assertive myself. . . . I was 35 years old when I got sick and usually it [starts] a lot earlier than that. I think that kind of threw him off."

Family doctors don't always have a lot of time. In a quick-fix world, physicians are often criticized for hasty diagnoses and prescribing of drugs (particularly for depression). So, if you're feeling rushed or ignored – and this applies to any professional – feel free to get a second opinion. If you're not getting better, try another GP or ask for a referral to a specialist.

Many specialists won't take on new patients without a referral. "In terms of the way our system is constructed," says Neasa Martin, former executive director of the Mood Disorders Association of Ontario and Toronto, "the GP is the most consistent, connected network of support."

Every GP should have the names and numbers of a couple of psychiatrists, psychologists, and other mental health professionals – people they've dealt with regularly and feel comfortable recommending. If those specialists can't see you promptly – and long waiting lists have, unfortunately, become the norm – your GP can provide interim care, often in consultation with a specialist.

In Canada, there's a growing emphasis on this kind of collaboration. Many doctors are becoming involved with something called "Shared Care" – a co-operative venture between the Canadian Psychiatric Association and the College of Family Physicians of Canada. This gives family practitioners the option of consulting with a psychiatrist about symptoms and treatment options. It's believed this model will be particularly useful in remote or underserviced areas, and with people who've found a GP – but not a psychiatrist – who speaks their first language.

The most common way of finding a psychiatrist in Quebec is through your nearest Centre local de service communautaire (CLSC). There are roughly 150 of these across the province; these agencies either have psychiatrists on staff or can find you one. (Most CLSCs also have links with other local mental health services.)

Your family doctor is a common place to begin your search for help

Psychiatrists

Like your GP, a psychiatrist has a degree in general medicine and has passed exams to become an MD. But the psychiatrist has then gone on to complete four additional years of specialist training and will have completed a residency at a psychiatric facility.

The psychiatrist you're referred to could be in private practice, or work at an out-patient clinic of a general hospital. (We'll talk about in-patient psychiatry later.) He or she – but most are still men – will be qualified both to prescribe drugs and do psychotherapy. If talk therapy is what you're after, there are any number of other professionals you can work with. Psychiatrists are the only therapists universally covered by provincial health plans; family doctors who practise psychotherapy are usually covered.

Consumers report that finding a good psychiatrist can be a major undertaking. In some regions of the country – and especially in rural communities – there simply aren't enough to go around. Psychiatrists are sometimes accused of devoting too much time to the so-called "worried well," at the expense of people with serious disorders.

For all these reasons, depending on where you live, you might have to wait several weeks, or travel some distance, before you actually get to sit in a psychiatrist's office. Then there are no guarantees you'll actually like the guy. Too often, consumers wait weeks or months to see someone, pinning their hopes for recovery on that crucial first visit, only to find they *don't* like him.

One strategy is to get yourself on several waiting lists at once. This can shorten the wait time, and improve your chances of finding someone you like. If you're expecting to have long-term contact with a psychiatrist, it's worth the initial effort to find the right match.

"If you can't form a relationship, there is no therapy," says Moira Mosher, a social worker who runs a telephone referral service for the CMHA. "If you're at odds with the psychiatrist, you're not going to get the help, or you're not going to accept it." She adds that most people can tell fairly quickly – in two or three sessions – if the fit is right.

Some people also find it helpful to bring a friend or family member along for support, especially to a first session. Someone who can advocate, ask questions, and gather information on your behalf.

What can you expect in that first session? The goal will be to confirm a diagnosis; all treatment flows from that. We asked Michael Myers, president of the CPA, what people have a *right* to expect from a psychiatrist during this stage. Dr. Myers's practice is devoted to doctors who themselves have mental disorders. And he answered in terms of his own approach. It's a thorough answer, based firmly in a biopsychosocial approach (encompassing possible biological, psychological, and social causes and treatments), so we'll quote it at length:

> *Say I think he or she has major depression. What I want to do is take a very good genetic, family history to find out if there's been any family members with a history of a mood disorder. I need to know his general medical health to make sure there aren't any physical factors contributing to his symptoms – thyroid disease or other . . . problems. I want to know about any medications or street drugs that he might be taking, and any previous depressions. I also want to know, of course, about his alcohol use. So a lot of that stuff is all in the area of biological psychiatry. . . .*
>
> *But then I want to have a very detailed developmental history on him. I want to know if his parents split up, for instance, when he was a child or adolescent. Whether or not he might have been abused, whether or not he might have had a learning disability. Whether or not he might have had some catastrophic [life event] that might have put him off-course for a while. So, all of the kind of psychological factors that might have contributed to his self-esteem, his personality development, things like that. . . .*
>
> *Now the sociocultural part is whether or not he's a member of an ethnic minority. . . . Did he grow up in poverty? . . . Religious persecution? Gay bashing? Things like that. Because it's the last part, the psychosocial part, that helps a lot in setting up your psychotherapy plan. So even if I conclude that this guy needs to go on an antidepressant, okay, that's fine. I'll monitor his mood. But I want to also get at any of the other stuff that's in his background.*

We should add that many people have told us they don't get anything like that kind of care. What they've seen, instead, are psychiatrists who ignore the psychosocial side and focus solely on biochemistry. One consumer who received this kind of treatment states emphatically, "I'm a person! I'm much more than biochemicals."

"In our province," says Dr. Myers, who practises in British Columbia, "one of the complaints about psychiatrists is that we don't do enough psychotherapy, that we are having to focus too much on the medication part of it. Either because of being busy or the psychiatrists are perhaps just so biologically oriented that they don't really function biopsychosocially."

Because of this, some people are turned off of psychiatry altogether. They want nothing to do with the "take-your-pills-and-see-you-later" approach. Psychiatrists are certainly not for everyone. But it's worth noting that within psychiatry, there is a *range* of approaches. Some doctors are more drug-oriented, others more interested in psychotherapy (see pages 158–62 for a description of the various kinds of psychotherapy practised); many will try to custom-blend the two. So it may take some time to connect with someone whose approach matches your own.

"There's very little consensus among health-care practitioners about how to treat the same problem," explains one mental health professional. "If you go to Dr. A, they may say [psycho]analysis is the route to go. If you go to Dr. B, they may say cognitive-behavioural therapy is what we should be doing. The third one will tell you it's a synaptic neurotransmitter problem and say, 'Here, take this pill.'"

And that's not a bad thing. That diversity presents options – one of which may mesh with your *own* view of what ails you.

Once a diagnosis is made, you should ideally be presented with a range of treatment options. These may include medication, psychotherapy, referral to a social worker or occupational therapist, all of the above, or none. That last option is not to be overlooked. Sometimes, the final assessment will be that no psychiatric treatment is required. Sometimes, distress has nothing to do with disorder.

The benefits and risks (including side effects) of each pro-
posed treatment should be clearly outlined and compared to
the benefits and risks of the alternatives – including the
option of no treatment at all. Your input is critical at this
stage; don't feel pressured into accepting treatment you're
uncomfortable with. Listen to your psychiatrist's recommendations, then go away and do some research. Read
widely, talk to other consumers, and consider your options.
Then, in consultation with your psychiatrist, make the
choices you feel will benefit you most.

Experienced consumers will tell you, it's essential to explain
your needs and opinions, and ensure that they're respected.
That applies to any doctor – psychiatrist or GP – no matter
how long you've been seeing them. Every therapeutic alliance
is a two-way street. That means you have the right to ask
questions and expect a thoughtful reply. It means you should
be treated in a respectful, sensitive, and supportive manner.

"I think it's really important for the consumer/patient to
demand a lot from their physicians and to challenge their
physicians to provide them with the kind of service that they
need to have," says Dr. Stan Kutcher, a clinical psychiatrist and
head of the Department of Psychiatry at Dalhousie University
in Halifax. "I think that traditionally the process has been a
different way, and I'm not in favour of that."

Something else to consider: doctors aren't always right.
Misdiagnosis, by family doctors *and* psychiatrists, is still far
too common. In one study by the Depressive and Manic-
depressive Association of Ontario, 60% of people surveyed
said they'd been misdiagnosed. The CMHA's B.C. Early
Intervention Study found nearly half of participants had, at
some point, been incorrectly diagnosed.

Because diagnosis is based on symptoms, it's an imprecise
science. Bipolar disorder, for example, can look like schizophrenia during a psychotic phase. In the early stages of
schizophrenia, a young withdrawn person may appear to be
suffering from depression. If more than one disorder is

involved – depression and anxiety, for example, or bipolar disorder and substance abuse – only one of them might be recognized and treated. In many provinces, substance-abuse and mental health services are completely separate entities, although efforts are underway to link the two more effectively.

For all of these reasons, if you're not satisfied with your initial diagnosis, you might want to consider a second opinion. This is *not* a betrayal on your part; doctors should accept this as your right. Unfortunately, many consumers choose to stay with their doctor, even if they're not getting better, out of a sense of loyalty.

Bear in mind, though, that recovery takes time. Drugs might need several weeks to take effect; psychotherapy usually takes longer. You and your psychiatrist should set specific goals, and a time frame by which they might be met. These can be assessed frequently, and if they aren't being met, new approaches can be pursued.

If medications are involved, your psychiatrist will oversee the regime, prescribing drugs, altering dosages and combinations, monitoring side effects, and ordering blood tests to determine therapeutic levels. Generally speaking, psychiatrists have far more expertise with psychotropic drugs than do family practitioners, including knowledge of their interactions with other medications.

Since medications are covered in Chapter 8, we'll focus now on psychotherapy. As we've said, not all psychiatrists practise it. But if the doctor you're seeing doesn't do psychotherapy, he or she should be able to refer you to someone who does.

Find someone you like and whose approach matches your own

Psychologists and Other Therapists

In most provinces, family doctors can practise psychotherapy. These GP-psychotherapists provide psychotherapy in their offices, either exclusively or as part of their general practice. Their numbers are growing and their services are covered by provincial health-care plans. Although most voluntarily take extra training in psychotherapeutic techniques, bear in mind that there is no requirement to do so. You may want to ask what experience or qualifications they have.

Psychologists are another option. They hold doctoral degrees, but are not medical doctors. Their specialty is the human mind – its nature, function, and influence on behaviour.

"We would approach the same issues as a psychiatrist, but from more of a psychosocial or a learning point of view," says Dr. John Service, executive director of the Canadian Psychological Association, "to help people change their attitudes or teach them new behaviours in order to rectify the situation or prevent the situation from occurring again."

There are three times as many psychologists as psychiatrists in Canada. In Quebec, a province with a greater emphasis on psychotherapy, the ratio is even higher. Although some psychologists take specialized courses in pharmacology, they are not permitted to prescribe drugs in Canada. They do, however, have greater training in psychotherapy than most GP-psychotherapists.

Unfortunately, psychologists who work in private practice are not currently covered by provincial health plans. Your private health-insurance plan might cover part or all of the costs, usually for a set number of visits. (Insurance companies may require a referral from a physician.) Some psychologists will offer sliding fee scales if you can't afford their usual rate.

Other professionals who provide psychotherapeutic services include social workers and psychiatric nurses, who can take additional training and/or apprenticeships in psychotherapy. They tend to work in hospitals or community agencies. But some do work in private practice, and again, those particular services are not covered by provincial health plans.

Your family doctor or psychiatrist should be able to refer you to any of these licensed therapists. Most professional associations also have telephone referral lines and will provide names of psychologists in your area (see Appendix). Support groups are good referral sources, too; staff and members are usually happy to share their own experiences and recommend people. But the best source is probably close friends and family who've used a therapist themselves.

"Don't be afraid to talk about it to somebody you trust," says Dr. Service. "And ask somebody you trust who might be of help. Because the best way to find a good psychologist is by word of mouth. So the first step is: don't be afraid to bring it up and ask."

One final warning. Anyone can hang a sign on their door saying "counsellor" or "therapist." The terms themselves have no licensing requirements attached to them. If you see someone whose training and qualifications are not apparent – either posted in an office or written on a business card – ask them about it.

As with psychiatrists, it's important to find someone you like and feel comfortable with, and whose approach to therapy meshes with your own. As we'll see, there are many types of psychotherapy, and figuring out what works for you can take some research.

"People, when they look for psychotherapy, often don't know what they're getting," says Zindel Segal, a psychologist with the Centre for Addiction and Mental Health (CAMH) in Toronto. "They could get a psychiatrist or a GP who does therapy and get anything from holotropic breathing to long-term psychoanalytic psychotherapy. . . . So consumers need to educate themselves around what they're looking for and knowing how to identify it."

Types of Psychotherapy
All psychotherapy involves talking to a professional. The idea is to build a relationship with the therapist – one that allows you to explore and resolve central issues in your life. You may not even know yet what those issues are, but the theory is that talking encourages self-understanding and discourages destructive behaviours and beliefs.

Psychotherapy has expanded hugely since the days of Freud, and there are now hundreds of techniques being practised. Many of the newer ones last weeks rather than years. And increasingly, as treatment becomes more refined and also more measurable, specific techniques are being tailored to specific disorders. In fact, research has proven that psychotherapy can have a physical effect, inducing measurable changes in the brain.

Psychotherapy helps with a wide range of disorders. Sometimes it works best on its own, sometimes in conjunction with drug therapy. Even with serious mental disorders, when medication is the primary treatment, psychotherapy can help people cope with the inevitable disruptions in daily life and self-esteem brought on by the diagnosis itself.

Kay Redfield Jamison, a psychiatrist who has bipolar disorder, eloquently describes her own need for therapy in her book *An Unquiet Mind*. "Lithium prevents my seductive, but disastrous highs," she writes, "diminishes my depressions, clears out the wool and webbing from my disordered thinking, slows me down, gentles me out, keeps me from ruining my career and relationships, keeps me out of a hospital, alive, and makes psychotherapy possible. But ineffably, psychotherapy heals. It makes some sense of the confusion, reins in the terrifying thoughts and feelings, returns some control and hope and possibility of learning from it all."

Psychotherapy isn't for everyone. It requires a commitment of time and energy. Time, because you have to show up week after week; energy, because talking can be challenging work. Some people find they're getting nowhere after months or years of sessions. Others find the experience overwhelming, emotionally draining.

But when it works, as one practitioner told us, "It's a very beautiful thing." People have told us psychotherapy changed – even saved – their lives, providing the kind of understanding and support found nowhere else in the system.

Some of the more common types of therapy include the following:

- *Psychoanalysis.* The stuff of Sigmund Freud, what people might wrongly assume all therapy to be. Lying on a couch, with the analyst out of sight, you are encouraged to "free associate," or talk about whatever comes to mind. The goal is to get into your unconscious mind – to become aware of the thoughts and feelings that began in childhood and now hide beneath the surface. The analyst's role is to listen non-judgmentally as you explore the relationship between your past and present. Traditionally, they provide minimal input, but this is changing; many modern analysts are more open to two-way communication. Psychoanalysis is a long-term undertaking, usually involving several sessions a week for several years.

- *Psychodynamic therapy.* This is similar to psychoanalysis, in that the focus is still on the unconscious, on exploring early childhood experiences, unresolved conflicts, and the ways these have shaped you in adult life. But you sit face-to-face with the therapist, who may provide more of his or her observations and insight. Therapy is usually less intensive, and may involve as little as one session per week.

- *Cognitive-behavioural therapy (CBT).* This is based on a simple premise: How you think affects how you feel. The goal is to break down those negative thought patterns that cause distress. First, you and the therapist figure out what those thought patterns are. This involves homework, writing down what you think in different situations. What automatically leaps to mind? For example, your boss praises you at work, but you instantly assume he doesn't mean it. The next step is to figure out if these thoughts are irrational. You look at the evidence behind your belief, and examine other explanations. (Maybe your boss is genuinely pleased with your work.)

  "A lot of what cognitive therapy does is look at ways of teaching people skills to deal with emotional upset," says Dr. Segal, who heads the Cognitive Behaviour Therapy Unit at CAMH, "so that they can find ways of preventing that upset from spiralling into a full-blown depression or a full-blown panic attack."

This therapy has proven effective for depression (with response rates comparable to antidepressants), panic disorder, obsessive-compulsive disorder, and generalized anxiety disorder.

- *Interpersonal therapy (IPT).* This is used mainly for depression. The idea is that if you improve your relationships, you'll also improve your mood. The first step is to identify the issue you want to address. That issue may be grief over a lost relationship; a role transition (for example, a mother whose child leaves home for university); interpersonal disputes (ongoing struggles with a spouse, friend, boss, or family member); or a more general problem with social functioning. Once you've figured out the central problem, you and the therapist work on thoughts, behaviours, and beliefs that can be adapted. As one IPT therapist notes, "Treatment success depends not just on understanding but on enacting life change." Recent research suggests IPT can also be effective with some other disorders, including bulimia.

These last two newer therapies tend to be brief – usually fewer than twenty sessions. But research demonstrates the benefits can be long-lasting, reducing relapses. IPT and CBT tend to be practised by psychologists; psychiatrists are more likely to practise psychoanalysis or psychodynamic psychotherapies.

The success of all these approaches depends on a relationship of trust and respect, and the sense that the therapist is on your side. It's important to feel you're being listened to, but not judged. And again, goal-setting is important; core issues should be identified early. Unlike those eternal therapy sessions depicted in old Woody Allen movies, psychotherapy is rarely a lifelong endeavour. Most people respond within a few months.

Group therapy (usually six to twelve people) may involve any number of therapeutic techniques. It's worth considering if you feel you may benefit from more than one opinion, and the support of others in similar circumstances. It's also cheaper than individual therapies.

> *A very wide range of proven psychotherapies exists. Learn which may be of maximum benefit in your specific case.*

Higher Support Services

For people with more chronic or severe symptoms, it may not be enough simply to see a physician or psychotherapist at their office. They may require, or want, higher levels of support.

Not so long ago, that meant just one option: hospital. Now, long-term hospitalization is considered a last resort, to be avoided whenever possible. Treatment in the community is considered to be less disruptive, and we now know people with serious disorders can thrive outside of hospital with appropriate supports. That applies even to people who've spent long periods in psychiatric institutions.

New Brunswick recently demolished its oldest psychiatric hospital, and former residents are now doing well in the community. Many of these people had spent years, even decades, on the inside.

"I never thought some of those people coming out would make it," says the director of a community mental health centre in Fredericton, "but in fact their needs have declined."

It's clear that most people with serious disorders can – and should – live in the community. Recent Canadian research confirms that even acutely psychotic individuals can be successfully treated at home, with adequate supports. This approach is cost-effective for government and preferable for many consumers. Receiving support at home – having the professional come to *you* – can be far more empowering than vice versa. (Some people, however, resent the intrusion and reject these services.)

There's a variety of options out there; some emphasize psychosocial supports, while others focus more on medication. We'll offer thumbnail sketches of a few of these services, most of which are tailored for the people deemed the "seriously mentally ill."

- *Mobile crisis units* can come to your home during a psychiatric crisis. People who staff these units are trained to assess the situation and determine a course of action. They're also skilled at dealing with a person who is suicidal or in psychosis, and can sometimes defuse an escalating emergency. Depending on the situation, these services can either prevent hospitalization or arrange for an admission. Units can be called by the individual in need or by family members (though some units will respond only with the permission of the person in crisis). While not universally available, these services are increasingly common and have been identified as a "best practice" – meaning the evidence shows they work.
- *Home visits* involve a professional developing a primary relationship with a consumer and checking in regularly. This person tries to offer assistance with many aspects of daily living, ranging from keeping an eye on symptoms to grocery shopping and budgeting – even alleviating loneliness. The most common model is known as "case management." Case managers help people improve their living skills and make the most of their personal strengths. Case management can be helpful not only for people living on their own, but as an added support for family members. Psychiatric nurses, social workers, and occupational therapists may also pay home visits. These professionals usually know the mental health system inside out and can help link clients with other community programs.
- *Assertive community treatment (ACT) teams* are affiliated with hospitals and include a psychiatrist, psychologist, psychiatric nurse, social worker, and occupational therapist. Members use their collective expertise to assist the

client in issues ranging from medication management to housing to employment. It's like an intensive version of case management, with a wider knowledge base at its disposal. Consumers supported by ACT teams are usually people with severe disorders who have a history of frequent hospitalization. Although team members often rotate their visits, one or two of them will usually develop a closer relationship with the client.

Unfortunately, these services can be difficult to track down. You're not likely to find "Mobile Crisis" or "Case Management" in your local phone book; you'll generally need to know the name of the service agency first. Doctors aren't always up on those names, so you may need to do some digging. Ask for names and numbers at your local hospital, CMHA office, community health centre, or provincial health ministry.

If these services aren't available, or if the situation worsens, you or your doctor may feel a hospital stay is necessary. But here, too, there may be alternatives available. There's a small but growing number of models ranging from crisis housing with strong medical support, all the way through to innovative places like Toronto's Gerstein Centre, a non-medical facility staffed by psychiatric consumer/survivors. Executive director Paul Quinn says the emphasis is on practical assistance and support.

"It's an alternative to [hospitalization] if people don't particularly want the kinds of interventions that are at a hospital," he says. "[We] try to give people an opportunity to resolve their own crisis and to see that they have the skills and abilities to do that."

If you feel you need a safe place to stay – but do not wish to go to hospital – check with your local CMHA or Mood Disorders Association. Although it's less likely in smaller cities, there may be other options near you.

In cases where the needs are greater, more intensive community supports may be helpful

Hospital

*"It was the most depressing experience of my lifetime.
The milieu on the ward was terrible. . . . I wouldn't go
back there."*

*"I thought it was a holiday, the most wonderful place in
the world."*

– B.C. Early Intervention Study

As these statements indicate, the range of hospital experiences is enormous. We've heard countless stories – good and bad – about stays on psychiatric wards. Some have found it a comforting and caring environment, while others have described it as coercive and callous. We know people who were desperate to get in, only to be told there were no beds, and others who were admitted against their will and were desperate to get out.

Entering a hospital is never pleasant. But entering a psych ward can be especially *un*pleasant. Some consumers feel a sense of failure or defeat, hopelessness or sorrow. Emotional responses vary depending on why and how people are admitted. "Some people eventually were relieved that they were getting some help," says Macnaughton of the B.C. Early Intervention Study. "But often the feeling of relief would be mixed with a feeling of trauma from being admitted in sometimes a rough way."

Generally speaking, there are two ways to be admitted. One is voluntary, the other involuntary.

Voluntary — There are a couple of ways to get yourself into hospital. One is to present yourself at Emergency and state your need for immediate help. You can do this at a psychiatric hospital or a general hospital.

These days, you're most likely to wind up at a general hospital. Psychiatric hospitals have been closed or downsized in most provinces, their services shifting towards people with serious and chronic disorders. Short-term care and crisis intervention have shifted to general hospitals, most of which now have psychiatric wards.

Statistics from the Canadian Institute for Health Information for 1995–96 reflect the very different roles these hospitals play. Eighty-five per cent of hospitalizations for mental disorder were in general hospitals, where the average length of stay was thirty-two days. In psychiatric hospitals, which accounted for the other 15%, the average length of stay was 261 days.

Getting admitted, in either kind of facility, can be difficult. There are simply fewer beds available nowadays.

"Gone are the days when someone says, 'I'm feeling sort of depressed, I think I'll sign myself into hospital,'" says social worker Moira Mosher.

Part of the difficulty is the nature of mental disorder itself. Staff at Emerg – more accustomed to treating fractured legs or heart ailments – can't see it, measure it, the same way they can X-ray a broken limb. And so they may underestimate, or fail even to realize, how much pain you are in. A common complaint is that mental health expertise is sorely lacking.

"The staff who work in emergency settings are not equally trained in how to deal with mental health crises as they are trained to deal with physical health crises," says B.C. Mental Health Advocate Nancy Hall.

If you show up at the wrong time, there may not be a psychiatrist or psychiatric nurse available. You may or may not be greeted with sympathy and respect. Your admission will depend on whether beds are available that day, and how critical your need is judged to be. In this kind of pressure-cooker atmosphere, people who show up voluntarily, requesting help, may be seen as less urgently in need.

"If the person is asking for help, there's a Catch-22 mentality," says Macnaughton. "If they're well enough to ask for help, they're not sick enough to deserve it." (A tale that once made the rounds in Ontario described a man being refused admission because he showed up with his suitcase. It he was "together" enough to pack his bags, went the story, then he wasn't ill enough to merit hospitalization.)

Many consumers report that they had to return several times before finally being admitted. You might want to have a friend or family member there to advocate on your behalf. But even then, there are no guarantees.

"Sometimes people have to go home and wait for a bed," says Mosher. "And sometimes they have to go to another hospital, because the hospital nearest to them doesn't have a bed."

One consumer in Macnaughton's survey resorted to desperate measures after being turned away. "The next time I came with a note that said 'I'm going to kill myself, and if you don't admit me it will be your responsibility.' It worked."

Macnaughton's advice is to keep trying, to "realize that if you think something is not quite right, you can't take no for an answer." But these days, that's easier said than done. This is where support networks can help. "In those kinds of situations, where they're getting their problems minimized . . . they have to turn to the local advocacy groups – the CMHA or Schizophrenia Society or Mood Disorders groups – because the knowledge about how to work the system is within those groups."

If you're too overwhelmed to make these calls yourself, ask a trusted friend or family member. Phone numbers are listed in the Appendix.

The second way to gain a voluntary admission is with the assistance of your family doctor or psychiatrist. Many physicians in private practice are affiliated with a hospital; they do consulting or clinical work there. They may have admitting privileges, or be able to pull some strings to find you a bed.

Once you *are* admitted, what happens on the inside can vary widely. There's usually a psychiatric examination, and an assessment to reach or confirm a diagnosis. Sometimes the friend or family member accompanying you will also be interviewed. Treatment plans vary; some emphasize medication, while others include psychotherapy, occupational therapy, group therapy, and social-work support.

A common complaint, in this era of cutbacks, is that hospitals do not keep people long enough. While that concern is understandable, research does not support the belief that longer hospital stays are somehow "better" for people.

"Length of stay is not related to client outcome," well-known U.S. health planner Dr. Trevor Hadley told a conference for mental health professionals. "There isn't a shred of evidence to demonstrate that being in a bed longer does anything good for you."

The problem is that many people leave hospital with no supports in place. This is where social workers come in. They may be able to help arrange for emergency or assisted housing, income assistance, or in-home visits from a psychiatric nurse once you are discharged from hospital. They should know of hospital day-programs and other support or self-help groups in your area. If you haven't met with a social worker in hospital, ask for an appointment.

Upon discharge, you should also be referred back to your GP or psychiatrist, who should be familiar with the circumstances of your hospitalization and with the treatment you've been receiving. If you do not have a regular physician, ask the hospital for a referral as part of your discharge plan.

> *Voluntary admissions are not as easy to obtain as in the past; your doctor may be able to help if you feel you need admission*

Involuntary — Somebody could write an entire book on this subject – on the intricacies and legalities of involuntary hospitalization from one province to the next. For our purposes, in *this* book, we will say that voluntary is always preferable, but involuntary hospitalizations are still common. More than half the people surveyed in the CMHA's B.C. study had been hospitalized against their will at least once.

Although mental health acts vary substantially in wording from province to province, they're all similar in one respect:

they all try to achieve a balance of rights. No small task, given the conflicting views on the topic.

People who call themselves "psychiatric survivors" often complain of terrible abuses they've suffered inside hospital walls. They associate involuntary hospitalization with coercion, force, cruelty. Many see involuntary hospitalization as a violation of fundamental human rights.

Many family members, however, have watched helplessly and repeatedly as loved ones deteriorated before their eyes. They've had hospitals turn them away, saying that the person doesn't meet the criteria for involuntary admission. They, too, believe a fundamental human-rights issue is at stake: the right to treatment.

The debate gets even more complicated when you throw wider public opinion into the mix. Alarmed by rare but high-profile crimes involving the mentally disordered, the public demands the right to safety, wants laws to ensure that someone who is potentially dangerous won't be wandering the streets.

"And the difficult thing about this debate is that all of those people are right," says lawyer Michael Bay, chair of the Consent and Capacity Board of Ontario and an authority on mental health legislation. "Every one of them is right. Therefore, the only way to make good law and good policy is to listen to all of them and attempt to achieve balance."

The Laws — Historically, there have been two dominant models of mental health legislation in Canada, models which attempt to achieve that balance in slightly different ways. One emphasizes what is often called the "best interests" of the person with the disorder, while the other puts more weight on their potential to pose a danger.

In mental health acts that stress dangerousness, people with a mental disorder who have harmed, are likely to harm, or have threatened to physically harm either themselves or others can be involuntarily hospitalized. Although acts like this contain other criteria, this is the *predominant* test for involuntary hospitalization.

Laws like these are often criticized by family organizations for being too narrow, because someone can be very unwell yet still fail to satisfy the criteria. We know one mother whose son, in a psychotic state, believed there was a conspiracy to poison him; he would consume only food that had been partially eaten, and therefore could not be poisonous. His mother saw him, day after day, scavenging in the garbage bin at a local McDonald's, eating scraps of burgers. And yet, because he was not truly posing a danger to himself or others, he likely would not have satisfied the criteria. Up until December of 2000, this was the way things were in Ontario.

Saskatchewan, in contrast, has for years used the other model of mental health law. Although it contains provisions regarding harm to self or others, the greatest weight is placed on "best interests": if it's believed the person is in need of treatment, is unable to *understand* their need for treatment, and is likely to suffer substantial mental or physical deterioration *without* treatment, then they can be involuntarily hospitalized. In the case of the young man mentioned above, he could be held against his will in Saskatchewan. (With the recent changes to Ontario's mental health act, he would likely now satisfy that province's criteria, as well.)

So every province is different, and the laws are subject to change. The best advice we can give – for both family members and consumers – is to know your rights under the law.

Generally, an involuntary committal happens in stages. The first stage is a short period of time – two or three days – during which your mental state will be assessed. After that assessment, depending on whether it's felt you satisfy the legal criteria for involuntary hospitalization, you may be released, or held for a longer period of time.

Every hospital should have a list of patient rights and hospital policies posted, or available upon request. In every province there is a procedure for appealing an involuntary committal. If you feel you are being held unlawfully, it is your right to appeal.

Many hospitals have rights advisers or patient-relations co-ordinators on site who will explain the appeals process. At the very least, the hospital should make available the phone numbers for local advocacy or consumer/survivor groups, who can inform you of your rights and avenues of appeal. Several provinces – including British Columbia, Alberta, Ontario, and New Brunswick – have advocacy offices set up specifically to help consumers with these and other issues.

It must also be noted that, in certain circumstances, things can get rough. Force is sometimes used to subdue an agitated or psychotic person. An actively suicidal or extremely aggressive patient may be locked in a "seclusion room," which is generally furnished with little more than a bed or mat on the floor.

The B.C. Mental Health Advocate's office receives complaints from mental health consumers across the province. About 20% of those complaints involve poor care or harsh treatment in hospital settings: people being locked in rooms with no sinks or toilets or without their clothes. "Some consumers feel they'd rather go to jail," says advocate Nancy Hall. "The services are better there." This is especially true, she notes, in small rural hospitals with inadequately trained staff.

"I've been needled and locked in side rooms and stuff," says Joan E. of Northern Ontario, "and I just can't handle them anymore. I just can't do it. Your best hope is to sleep, cooperate, be quiet – and get out." Conversely, some consumers credit involuntary hospitalizations with restoring their sanity – even saving their life.

The length of time someone is involuntarily hospitalized depends, as you might guess, on how long they meet the legal criteria. Once there's enough improvement, the status changes to "voluntary" – whereupon the person is free to leave (or stay, if needed).

The laws governing involuntary hospitalization are very technical and don't make easy reading. So it's important to find a "plain language" guide to involuntary hospitalization laws in your province. (These are often published in several languages.)

Having that knowledge can be a powerful tool in cases where you disagree – either as a consumer or a family member – with a doctor's decision. If you know the criteria cold, you have every right to discuss or debate this important decision with the person making it.

"In this world, when you go to a professional – a lawyer, a travel agent, a nurse," Bay says, "your best defence is to know more about the subject than them and to teach them."

It may require a little looking, but often your local hospital, CMHA office, Schizophrenia Society chapter, or Legal Aid office will know where you can find one of these easy-to-read guides. These booklets generally include information on the appeals process as well.

Find a "plain language" guide to your mental health legislation

Involuntary Treatment — In some provinces, involuntary hospitalization and involuntary treatment go hand in hand. If you're ill enough to be admitted against your will, the thinking goes, you're ill enough to be treated against your will. But not always. Sometimes the two are treated separately – even covered by separate legislation.

The laws vary so widely across the country it's impossible to encapsulate them here, but few people are neutral on this topic. Some consumers express tremendous relief at being freed from a psychotic episode.

"The vast majority of people who are involuntarily treated are grateful afterwards," says one New Brunswick psychiatrist. "The vast majority say, 'Don't wait so long next time.'"

Others, however, would not share that view. Forced treatment can involve being put in restraints or held down by people much larger and stronger than you. It can feel more like punishment than treatment. People who have previously endured physical or sexual abuse can find it extremely traumatic;

some, in fact, have described it as being worse than rape.

There's also the fact that individual doctors have their own views. As a Canadian Psychiatric Association position paper points out, "Some psychiatrists are more permissive, others more authoritarian in their approach to treatment."

It's not an easy topic. Nor is there an easy way for a clinician to know how a person will respond to involuntary treatment. Will they be grateful afterwards? Or will they be scarred by the experience?

Family members as well as doctors face this dilemma. In cases where the person is deemed "incapable" – meaning they can't weigh options rationally – a spouse, close family member, or public trustee may be called upon to make the decision in the best interests of the patient. But how can we know what those best interests are?

One potential way of clarifying those interests is for the consumer to state them explicitly during a period when they are of sound mind, capable of fully foreseeing their ramifications. Though the language can differ, it's often referred to as a "prior capable wish" – and such wishes have been ruled valid by Canadian and U.S. courts. (The concept, very similar to that of a Living Will, is also supported by the Canadian Medical Association.)

Lawyer Anita Szigeti, chair of the Ontario Mental Health Legal Committee and a consumer/survivor advocate, says a typical prior capable wish might be worded as follows:

> No matter how depressed/manic/psychotic or otherwise mentally ill I may become without the administration of ECT [electroconvulsive therapy], I still wish to express now – while I have the mental capacity to do so – that under those circumstances should I ever again become ill, I do not wish to receive ECT.

Conversely, a prior capable wish could state that you want to be treated as early as possible during a psychotic episode, no matter *what* you say while psychotic. Although these desires can be expressed verbally, lawyers suggest they may be more obvious, and more likely to be respected, if they are written. It's also a good idea to have a statement witnessed, preferably by two people. Give your physician a copy, and request that it be added to your clinical chart.

Other legal options to explicitly convey your capable wishes are also available. If you wish to appoint a specific *individual* to make decisions on your behalf (should you become incapable), there are ways to do that. In Ontario, for example, the Ministry of the Attorney General publishes a booklet containing forms that you can use to make a Power of Attorney for Personal Care, letting you designate someone to make your treatment decisions if you become incapable. The same booklet also contains a form that you can use to make a Power of Attorney for Property, allowing you to authorize someone you trust to handle your financial affairs. In British Columbia, the new Representation Agreement Act – which became law in 2000 – allows you to take similar steps.

If any of the above options appeal to you, discuss them with a lawyer to ensure you fully understand their legal power – and that the wording satisfies your provincial laws. Although there is no guarantee these will be legally binding in *all* conceivable circumstances, prior capable wishes and powers of attorney are a proactive way of increasing the likelihood you'll receive the care you desire.

Not every province has legislation spelling out the legal power of your capable wishes. New Brunswick, for example, is an exception. Even there, however, some consumer/survivors have had their competent written desires for treatment respected by physicians.

> *Should you become incapable, legal tools can help ensure that your competent wishes are respected*

THE "INFORMAL" SYSTEM

So far, we've been talking about the "formal" medical system. But there's another world of support out there – one that hundreds of thousands of Canadians swear by. This informal system can be as casual as a drop-in centre where you can enjoy a coffee and relax, or as structured as a program designed to get you back to work. Many consumers report that this other system helps them as much as, if not more than, the formal system.

Self-help

Self-help groups offer a place to go where you'll always be welcomed, respected, and listened to. The goal is to provide support and information that the rest of the system overlooks. For some people, these groups are the first point of contact with the mental health system, while others only discover this support network years after being diagnosed.

Some groups are organized around specific disorders; others cast a wider net. Some include or are oriented toward family members; others are exclusively for consumers. The main national self-help organizations are the Canadian Mental Health Association (CMHA), the Schizophrenia Society, the Mood Disorders Association (MDA), and the National Network for Mental Health. In Quebec, one of the most prominent groups is the Alliance for the Mentally Ill (AMI-Quebec).

But there are many, *many* other support groups across the country – helping a whole range of consumers, from people with eating disorders, to victims of torture. Some groups are run for – and by – gays, lesbians, youth, and ethnocultural minorities. There are even, in many larger cities, "survivor" groups for people who feel psychiatry has harmed, rather than helped, them.

One of the foundations of self-help is the support-group meeting, where people can discuss what's happening in their lives in a structured and safe environment. It offers a unique kind of support – the type no drug or doctor can provide.

"You're not just talking to a doctor or a nurse or a therapist whose business it is to treat you," says Bill Ashdown of the Mood Disorders Association of Canada. "You are talking to somebody who has gone through the process, and who has been through the same situation that you're in – who has walked the walk and talks the talk."

There's tremendous comfort in listening to other people's stories, in discovering that your own experiences have been shared by many. There's hope in talking to people who've recovered; solace in meeting someone who's feeling just like you.

"At the end of the meeting," says Ashdown, "you'll often find people who – in this particular part of their lives – they're bosom buddies. They may be strangers in other regards, but they have this tangible connection. And that support is enormously valuable. You can't put a price on it, because these are enormously isolating illnesses."

Self-help organizations also offer practical information and support. Some provide books, videos, magazine articles, even referral services. All of them provide the wisdom of fellow consumers. People relate their own experiences and what they have learned about the system. They talk about drugs, doctors, therapy, alternative treatments, relationships – you name it. And they discuss it all in very frank terms. It's what one support-group director calls the "guerrilla guide to the system that you're not going to get from any health-care professional or any brochure."

With one quick phone call you can find out about the resources close to you. "If someone calls and asks, 'Is there something around in my county?' we'll scan our directory and try to hook them up," says Jean-Pierre Galipeault, programs manager of Nova Scotia's Self-Help Connection. "If nothing exists and you're interested in starting something, we'll help you."

Most self-help organizations also run programs of their own. The CMHA, for example, has projects to assist with housing or employment. The Mood Disorders Association regularly has meetings for family members of those with depression or bipolar affective disorder. The Schizophrenia Society frequently has guest speakers who work at the cutting edge of schizophrenia research. And the National Network for Mental Health is currently working on a number of employment initiatives.

Self-help programs result in measurable benefits. In 1997, the Health Systems Research Unit at the Clarke Institute of Psychiatry reviewed the scientific literature on self-help. In a report called "Best Practices in Mental Health Reform," the unit concluded that such programs are associated with:

- reduced hospitalization
- reduced use of other mental health services
- increased knowledge, information, and coping skills
- greater self-esteem, confidence, and sense of well-being
- greater feeling of "being in control"
- and stronger social networks and support.

These organizations have national, provincial, and local offices. In our Appendix, we've listed all the provincial headquarters; they can refer you to your closest local chapter.

Research has shown that self-help has measurable benefits. Many consumers feel it is critical to their well-being.

Clubhouses

These tend to be used by people with serious and persistent disorders; people often unemployed and marginalized due to their condition. Or, more accurately, marginalized due to the way society *perceives* their condition.

The goal of a clubhouse, in mental health lingo, is "psycho-social rehabilitation" (or PSR). The emphasis is on abilities rather than limitations. The concept – and reality – is that everyone has skills, regardless of the nature of their disorder.

"We support people to go back to work, to go back to school, to have meaningful participation in whatever way they desire," says Nancy Beck, program manager at Connections Clubhouse in Halifax. "Basically, what we do is provide a meaningful place for people to be supported, to move forward with their lives into the community." Beck says that approach is vastly different from the one traditionally taken with consumers, who find "their whole lives have been medicalized. And I think what clubhouses do is to break that mould and look more broadly at individuals and their capacities and help them move forward."

A less structured model is something called a drop-in. As the name implies, it's a casual place for consumers to visit. Some drop-ins offer meals and planned activities, others are basically a place to have a coffee and some conversation. Though their benefits may be less measurable than those of a clubhouse, drop-ins alleviate the tremendous isolation often felt by people with persistent mental disorders. There is an unconditional acceptance, a feeling of belonging.

"It's helped me stay out of the hospital," says Brenda M., who lives in Atlantic Canada. "It's a major, major support group for me, and I don't know what I'd ever do without it. This has literally been my lifeline."

These services do not always contain the words "drop-in" or "clubhouse" in their title (for example, Saskatoon's Crocus Co-op or Hamilton's Friendship Centres), so you may have a tough time finding them in your local phone book. Again, your local chapter of the CMHA, MDA, or provincial health ministry should know what's around.

Distress Lines
Open your phone book.

Generally, on the very first page, you'll find a number for a local distress or crisis line. Dial that number, and you'll reach a real person.

Many Canadians who've used these lines appreciate the anonymity involved. A deep or troubling issue can be discussed in a comforting atmosphere of trust and respect. The vast majority of those who answer the phones are highly trained volunteers. You get the sense they are listening to you because they *care*, not because they're being paid to. They're there to help, and they know the territory.

"People often call us because they don't know who to call," says Howard Kravitz of the Distress Centres of Ontario. "We're really the gateway to the system."

Support for Women
It's often said that women use mental health services twice as often as men. And yet those services often overlook the unique needs and experiences of women.

Women, for example, are more likely to experience poverty, discrimination, sexual harassment, and physical, sexual, or emotional abuse. They're more likely to be raising children on their own. And even if they're not single, they're more likely to carry the emotional and caregiving burdens of the family. (Research shows that marriage is a "protective factor" against mental disorder for men, but not for women.)

It sounds obvious: if you're in an abusive relationship, or raising your children alone and in poverty, pills alone will not restore you to full health. But professionals don't always address this simple truth.

"Psychiatrists and doctors might see women more, but they're not really addressing what women are coming to see them about," says Miriam Russell, who facilitates the Keele Street Women's Group, a Toronto support program for women with mental health problems. "They seem to tune out to all of this."

Most cities have services for women who've been abused. But often they're not well-integrated with mental health services. Pat Fisher is a trauma therapist and researcher. She suggests that if you have both mental health problems *and* are being, or have been, abused, you might try the women's agencies first. They specialize in dealing with the trauma arising from abuse, but you can ask them to provide help for your mental disorder too. But if you go to the mental health system for help, says Fisher, and say "I need somebody who understands trauma," you're probably less likely in most jurisdictions to find somebody who really understands the issues.

Women-only services are slowly starting to appear in larger cities. These include support groups, transition houses, and therapy centres for women with mental disorders. In Toronto, the Centre for Addiction and Mental Health (CAMH) has a new twenty-two-bed in-patient hospital unit designed specifically for women.

"The goal is to provide a very safe environment for women," says psychiatrist Brenda Toner. "For them to feel that they could be nurtured."

Women-centred or feminist therapy is another option. The focus is not only on diagnosis and symptoms, but also on increasing a woman's strength, confidence, and control over her environment. An increasing number of therapists in private practice are taking this approach.

Dr. Toner recommends that women exploring these issues also develop their own support networks. "If you do this in isolation, if you have new ideas, it can be crazy-making. So you really need to find other people, and especially women, who may understand or validate or share some of the concerns that you have."

The Keele Street Women's Group, run by the CMHA, is a good example. The group plans outings, activities, and is a safe place to talk. "The key word for this group is respect," one member says. "We all respect each other."

Some mental health services deal specifically with the needs of women

Multicultural Support

Research shows that your cultural background will influence the treatment you receive. You're less likely to get care, for example, if you don't speak English. You're much less likely to be referred to a specialist if you're a new immigrant.

And, conversely, if you do see a mental health professional, your cultural background may be considered unimportant. A frequent complaint is that mental health services are based on middle-class Western values and concepts of health and family.

"They [the medical profession] do not try to understand our ways," one consumer told the CMHA's "Hear Me Now" study. "It is difficult for us to trust them when they make no effort to understand us. Of course the way we handle this is unique – because we are unique."

That applies to the world of research, too. Drug trials, for example, have traditionally been conducted on white males; it's assumed the findings apply to everyone else. Research by Dr. Morton Beiser, who heads CAMH's culture, community, and health studies program, suggests this may be a false assumption.

"White males absorb antipsychotic medication – at least the particular one that we were dealing with, which was Haldol – at a much lower rate than women or than Chinese men," Dr. Beiser says. "So that means the white males may require higher doses of the medication."

People of Asian descent may suffer more side effects, or require lower dosages. But Dr. Beiser notes that many doctors are unaware of these differences.

Race may also play a role in diagnosis. Research suggests, for example, that white psychiatrists are more likely to diagnose a black patient with schizophrenia than they would a white patient with similar symptoms.

For all these reasons, in an ideal world you would make sure you found a mental health professional from your own cultural background, who spoke the same language. In the real world, this may not be possible, even in larger cities.

So you may need to be more assertive in your requests or demands for care. You may need to push doctors to understand your own perspective on mental health and treatment. And you may need to find a translator or advocate, preferably someone with mental health training, who can come to appointments with you. Ethno-racial community agencies can help with this. They may also provide counselling, and connect you with culturally sensitive mental health services.

"No matter what group you're working with, whether it's a particular ethnic group that's European or one of Canada's many minorities, it's very critical to use a culturally congruent approach," says George Renfrey, a psychologist of aboriginal descent. "And particularly one that is at least cognizant of the belief system."

The Western medical model is notoriously single-minded; there's little emphasis on spirituality or on holistic approaches to care. Whether it's Ayurvedic medicine, acupuncture, sweat lodges, or prayer, we encourage you to seek the kinds of treatment that match your own notions of mental health.

LYNDA'S STORY

In a few weeks I will be turning seventeen, and while most teenagers my age are thinking about going to college and hanging out with their friends, I am worrying about whether or not I will be alive next year to celebrate another birthday. Almost a year and a half ago I was diagnosed with anorexia nervosa. I was admitted into the Hospital for Sick Children eating disorder program in Toronto, Ontario, and forced to gain weight. That was the most traumatic experience I have ever gone through, and as a result of that I have been hospitalized seven more times within the past year.

I have tried to fight the hospital's so called "treatment" numerous times, and I have become a master at cheating the scale, both in and out of hospital, but there is only so much a person can try to hide before their whole lie falls apart. I remember lying in a hospital bed, attached to a cardiac monitor and an IV, pumping fluid into my dehydrated body. All I could think about was how much weight I was going to gain and how fat I was going to be. It hadn't occurred to me that I could have died at any minute from dehydration, starvation, or a heart defect. I would rather have died than gain the weight needed to get out *of hospital. I remember forcing myself to do hundreds and hundreds of sit-ups, push-ups, and leg lifts a day. I remember trying my best to hide any and all food; to me food was better in any place other than my mouth. Out of desperation, I actually became quite creative with hiding my food. It got to the point that even if I could spare a crumb from entering my mouth, I somehow felt better inside.*

Many people ask me how this all started. I wish this were a "once upon a time" story (one where in the end I could say, "and we all lived happily ever after"). But it isn't. If I had to speculate, find the "once upon a time" when it all began, I wouldn't know where to start. Some people say it's genetic or inherited, others believe it is learned from the media. I think all those factors contributed to my illness; it's hard to pinpoint an exact cause.

I was always a quiet kid, not very outgoing or social. Sometimes I felt like I had so much to say, but no one to tell it to. I was always very clean, overly concerned about "contracting germs." I had weird rituals, which I now know are related to obsessive-compulsive disorder. From early on in my childhood, I often felt that my mom played the role of both my parents. She was someone I could rely on, and sometimes I felt like she was the only one. I must admit I was, and still am, a worrywart; I worry about even the littlest things. I aimed at trying to please my parents, but no matter what I did I always felt like a failure. I cared what others thought of me more than what I thought about myself; somehow I thought that if people liked me, maybe I could learn to like myself. I always felt like nobody liked me. I had low self-esteem and often compared myself to others who did better than me, which made me hate myself more. And yet I managed to put on a happy face for everyone, when inside I was sinking into a depression.

I never paid much attention to my weight. As a child I ate what I wanted, when I wanted it. It wasn't until my last year of elementary school that I became "aware" of my weight. I don't know what changed, but I felt as though people would like me more if I was just a little thinner. I told myself that if I was thinner I would be happier. I started to exercise, I began counting fat grams and limiting my fat intake, and I decided to refrain from eating anything after eight o'clock. I slowly began losing weight. I didn't feel any different, however, and most importantly, I didn't feel any happier.

A few months later, I got my wisdom teeth taken out and I was in immense pain. For two days I was unable to eat much of anything. I became very weak and dizzy, I couldn't even bring myself to stand up or walk around. I sat on the couch all day watching the Food Network. I had lost four pounds over the previous two days! I felt like I had control. For a moment I felt a sense of happiness, like I had just won the Olympics. I felt that in order to succeed I had to continue my quest for "perfection"; I had to continue to starve myself. Little did I know that I was digging myself deeper and deeper into my own grave. This was the beginning of my ongoing struggle.

As a result of being in and out of hospital, I missed a whole year of school. I went back this September, and I have finally realized how much I have missed as a result of my illness. Within the last year, it seems like all my friends and classmates have matured and moved on with their lives, something I have not been able to do. Sometimes I wish I could be like a "normal" teenager, interested in music, friends, and just plain having fun. Instead I have to spend the climax of my teenage years alone, obsessing over calories and food. If I could turn back the clock to the exact point where I first unconsciously decided to start losing weight, I would definitely change the path I took. I would give up my whole life if I could take away all the pain I have caused my family.

A lot of people don't understand eating disorders, including some of the doctors I have met that specialize in the field. They assume that eating will magically cure the illness. Their ignorance, along with my determination to keep the eating disorder, has kept me from receiving the help I need. I am certain that if I had received the proper treatment when I was first diagnosed a year and a half ago, my current situation would be a lot different now.

It has been about a month since I left the hospital (for the eighth time). I am now searching for the help that I so desperately *hope for, but do not want. Although every day is a struggle, I am managing to stay afloat. I don't know how long this will last, and I cannot predict when or if I am ever going back into hospital. The thought of having to go back sends shivers up my spine. I like to think of myself as an injured bird, unable to fly and left behind by my flock. Although I am optimistic, no one can predict when I will catch up or if I'll ever fly again.*

CHAPTER SEVEN

Giving Help

"Mood disorder is a trip I would rather not take. When it happens, all I ask is that you understand I'm not a voluntary tourist."

"If there was a way to survive what I was going through as a person and as a wife, I could only find it with others who appreciated that we were normal human beings with ordinary aspirations and sorrows, and extraordinary burdens in living with mental illness."
— from You Are Not Alone, *a handbook by the Mood Disorders Association of Metropolitan Toronto*

Someone you know – a friend, family member, or colleague – has a mental disorder. What's your first reflexive response? Do you recoil in fear? Offer comfort and support? Avoid the issue altogether?

Whatever you say or do – even if you say or do nothing – your response will make a difference. It will have a direct impact on someone's welfare. The authors know this from personal experience. And we know it from speaking with lots of consumers, family members, and mental health professionals.

If that responsibility sounds daunting, it needn't be. Just look at the quotations above. They don't ask for much.

In our own case, reactions varied widely. Close friends and family were tremendously supportive, and made a huge difference in our daily lives. They may not have always known precisely what to say or do, but they cared, and we knew it. They helped in a couple of very basic ways. First, they issued no blame or judgment. And second, they assumed that Scott would fully recover. That kind of mindfulness is all too rare, we've learned.

From further afield, responses were mixed. Some people stuck around; others stayed away, in particular, the whole group of friends and colleagues we'd known in Moscow. From their quarter, the silence, as the saying goes, was deafening. We received not a single phone call, card, or letter; five years later, we still haven't heard from any of them.

We've heard this from many consumers: it's that wider circle of friends and associates that tends to clear out. Still, it hurts. Silence is a peculiar brand of rejection. Live with it long enough, and you assume you're disliked or disgraced, ridiculed or judged. If you know someone in mental distress, and are wondering whether to reach out, know this: it's always better to say or do *something* than nothing. Your efforts, large or small, will be remembered. They will help.

When someone is physically ill or injured – breaks a leg, has a heart attack, comes down with flu – we all know what to do. We send cards and flowers, make hospital visits, supply pots of soup. With mental disorder, it somehow gets more awkward. People don't know what to say, how to help.

In fact, there are plenty of ways to be supportive. And that's what this chapter is about. People's needs will vary according to their personality, circumstances, and diagnosis. There is no one foolproof, perfect method. But in speaking with consumers and family members, we have seen some common themes emerge – helpful first steps that most of us can take.

EDUCATE YOURSELF

This will help you as much as the person you're aiming to support. First, you can examine your own beliefs. Do you think "the mentally ill" are somehow lesser human beings? More violent? Less intelligent? Is it their own fault? Yours? We all have misconceptions; education helps us overcome them, replace them with facts.

There's lots of information out there, but finding it can be tough. Mental health professionals don't always provide the kind of basic, practical information people need. Libraries, bookstores, Internet sites, and support groups are all good resources. Read widely and talk to as many people as you can.

Even if you aren't a close family member, education is important. Armed with information, you'll be less likely to ask dumb questions, say the wrong thing, cause offence. You'll know that if your depressed friend can't get out of bed some mornings, he's not merely being lazy. You'll learn that your colleague's panic attacks or your cousin's delusions aren't something they can just "get over."

Becoming informed shows you cared enough to learn. And it engenders genuine empathy. Once you understand the disorder – its symptoms, treatment, and possible causes – you'll come a lot closer to understanding what the person's going through. Trust us, your efforts will be appreciated.

For close family members, there's a tremendous relief that comes with cracking open a book and finding a description of the very symptoms your loved one has displayed. The diagnosis becomes more than just a frightening word; the disorder takes shape, and things start to make sense.

Education also helps family members deal with "the system." Mental health professionals respect informed questions and input.

The danger of becoming informed, however, is that you might think you know what's best for your friend or family member. You're *sure* that if they just took their medication, or visited their doctor regularly, everything would be just fine. If this sounds like you, read on . . .

HAVE RESPECT

It sounds so simple, so *obvious*, but in fact it's really hard to do. Maybe the hardest thing of all. And that is to respect someone's choices, even when you're convinced they're wrong.

A daughter who won't take her meds, a husband who refuses to see a doctor, a mother who's behaving strangely but denies she's unwell: these are the most common problems raised at family support groups. And the ones with the fewest solutions. Because the painful truth is this: you can't *make* someone do what you decide is right.

Arguments don't help; yelling or criticizing will not change minds. In fact, high levels of what's called "expressed emotion" – critical, hostile, or overly emotional attitudes – are associated with higher relapse rates for some disorders.

So, know that you can't "fix" things, or save someone. What you *can* do is propose options, try to understand their choices, and respect their right to make them. Denial is typical with some disorders; admitting a need for help is a scary business. With time – and often, unfortunately, a worsening of symptoms – denial usually gives way to acceptance. But consumers need to do this in their own time.

Sometimes, too, the disorder causes what's known as "lack of insight," especially during psychosis; the person has no idea anything's wrong, and rejects all evidence to the contrary. ("Lack of insight" is a contentious phrase; some feel psychiatrists use it any time a consumer rejects a diagnosis, even when that rejection may be reasonable.)

Whatever the case, you are free to make suggestions and explain your reasons for concern. You can offer encouragement, support, and information – books, pamphlets, names of doctors. But always with the understanding that the person might not use them.

"I always say to people, 'If you chase them, they will run away,'" says one mental health professional who works with families. "Stop chasing. I know that in the long run, if the situation is to improve, it's because the person's willing to start to take some ownership of the illness."

So respect choices. But also respect the very real pain associated with disorder. Advice that doesn't fully acknowledge that pain is disrespectful.

"I very much appreciate it if people don't say, 'Snap out of it,'" one man who suffers from depression told us, "because I've already given myself that lecture so many times."

Cheer up, grow up, keep your chin up, stop exaggerating, don't feel sorry for yourself, these are unhelpful forms of advice. In fact, advice, however well-intentioned, is often unhelpful.

"If you give advice and it's good, then *you're* responsible for their wellness. If you give advice and it's bad, they are angry with you," says Neasa Martin, former executive director of the Mood Disorders Association of Ontario and Toronto. "If you give them advice and it's good and they don't take it, you are angry with them. . . . So when you find yourself giving advice a lot, shut up! It's not helpful."

Much better – and more appreciated – is plain old listening.

LISTEN

"We don't know how to not say anything. We think we have to solve the problem. All they want is for us to listen."

This is a voice of experience. Doris Sommer-Rotenberg had a son with bipolar affective disorder who died of suicide. "People ask me what advice would I give. I say listen. Accept the way they feel. Just the listening and accepting. You know, our instinct is to say, 'Oh, you can't feel that way.' And that doesn't help."

It's a refrain oft-repeated by consumers. They want their feelings acknowledged rather than dismissed.

"Just being there, saying, 'I care, I'll listen,'" one woman told us when asked how people can help most. "Even if they don't understand, they can just listen."

Think about the worst time in your life. A divorce, a serious injury, a death in the family. In times of distress, we all need the same thing: supportive listeners who can share our burden.

This is doubly so with *mental* distress, because stigma is so widespread, and genuine sympathy so rarely offered. If you listen openly – without fear or judgment – you'll be a welcome exception to the rule.

Former federal finance minister Michael Wilson often emphasizes the importance of listening. He also lost a son to suicide. And since Cameron's death, Wilson has tried to raise awareness by sharing his story. During a recent presentation, Wilson described how Cameron felt unable to talk about his depression, fearing people couldn't possibly understand. Wilson believes that fear was likely a contributing factor in his death.

"It's important to feel that it's okay to talk about the illness," Wilson said. "In fact, it's more than okay. It's essential."

Listening will help you, too. Your friend or family member can explain what they've endured, describe how they're feeling. And that leads to true understanding – something all the books in the world can't give you.

> *Listening helps the person unburden – and helps* you *understand*

FOCUS ON THE WHOLE PERSON

The most common message we heard from consumers was this: treat me normally. Treat me the way you always have, the way you would any other human being.

Again, the broken-leg analogy is useful. As a friend, family member, or colleague, you sympathize with the pain. You accommodate the limitations caused by the injury. But you assume the person remains fundamentally unchanged. It's the same with mental disorder.

"If you used to get mad at us when we did something, you can still get mad at us," one consumer told us, chuckling.

Likewise, if you used to enjoy a meal together, a walk, a movie, or a ball game, you can still share these activities. In fact, they are a crucial part of the recovery process. As social worker Kate Kitchen notes, a person with a disorder "is healthy and capable in many other ways. Focus on the whole person."

Even when someone's in hospital, it's important to normalize the experience as much as possible. It's easy to assume they want to be left alone until they're better. This is rarely true. In fact, our own fears keep us away from the hospital. But think about the message you send by staying away. Your visit may not be a cheery one; it may even be very brief. But your presence will count. Bring food and presents, send flowers and cards. Encourage others to do the same.

"You can actually ask people, because this is really important," one family member says. "Ask friends to show up, even if they may be uncomfortable." When her brother is in hospital, she brings her children along for visits. "He loves it," she says. "Children are the great equalizer."

View the person as an individual – not a disorder

FOR THOSE CLOSEST

Family members (and by that we mean anyone with intimate ties) have, in this era of cutbacks, become the frontline workers of the mental health field. It's often confusing, stressful, draining work. The odds seem stacked against you. You want what's best for your loved one, but aren't sure what that is. Where to turn for help? How to offer it in turn?

If this describes your own experience, you're certainly not alone. One CMHA study, called "Hear Me Now," asked more than a thousand family members to describe their experiences with the mental health system. The responses were a litany of frustrations and unmet needs. As one participant stated, "I had so many questions, and nobody had any answers."

Family members need supports of their own – supports that recognize *their* suffering – and often the system fails to provide them. Whether you're a spouse, parent, sibling, son, or daughter, you ride the emotional roller coaster with your family member. You suffer in different ways. But you suffer nonetheless.

"How I felt when I first encountered manic depression in my family," one father writes in the handbook *You Are Not Alone*. "*Bewildered* because I was in a quandary. *Confused* because I could make no sense of it. *Shocked* because I grovelled in fear. *Ignorant* because I knew absolutely nothing about the illness."

A mother writes in the same handbook: "A whole new world, unthought of and unwanted, opened up. There is the uncertainty as to how to behave toward this family member who is acting in such an unusual way, what to tell our neighbours and friends, how the rest of the family will react."

Mental disorder has a nasty tendency to divide families. Communication breaks down, dysfunction sets in. Marital conflict and divorce are far more common when one spouse has a disorder. One study found that depression, for example, had a far worse impact on marriages than did cardiac illness or rheumatoid arthritis.

But it doesn't have to be that way. With appropriate information, support, and planning, families can and do stay strong.

Here are some coping strategies, drawn from the wisdom of family members and professionals who work with them, and from our own experience.

Reducing Stress
Research shows that stressful environments can have an adverse effect on many disorders. "It is becoming increasingly apparent that a supportive, nonstressful social environment is important in sustaining remissions," one study of major depression concluded.

So, reducing stress will help your family member. It will help you, too. The irony, of course, is that mental disorder *creates* stress; when symptoms are severe, entire households can be overcome with it. But with time, experienced family members learn to adapt.

"When the diagnosis came for us, it changed our family life dramatically," one man told a recent meeting of family members. "We have learned as a family to go with the flow, to live in as stress-free an environment as possible."

So how do you get to that stage? First, acknowledge that you can't do everything. You can't, for example, treat your loved one's symptoms or serve as therapist; a trained professional should assume these roles. The best you can do is help your family member find the support he or she needs, and encourage them to use it. This will lower everyone's stress levels.

You can also learn, in time, to separate the person from the disorder. To do this, you need to know the symptoms well. And when those symptoms involve hurtful words or actions, blame the disorder, not the person. It's normal to feel angry or frustrated at times, but remind yourself that these symptoms are beyond the control of your family member. "Keep telling yourself that, and telling yourself the crisis will pass, and there is a tomorrow," advises one family member.

Experienced family members learn not to take things personally when presented with behaviour they would normally not tolerate. They disengage themselves from the symptoms of the disorder.

"They have to create a distance from the illness, but not from the person with the illness," says Dr. Sylvia Geist, past-president of the Schizophrenia Society of Canada. "If the illness is overwhelming, you need to stand back and say, 'I need to find ways of dealing with the illness but not reject the person I love.'"

Family members can also set boundaries, deciding for themselves which behaviours they simply cannot accept, and what consequences will follow if the behaviours continue. Calmly explain these behaviours and consequences, and why they're important to you.

At this and every other stage, it's helpful to stay positive – to state what you want to happen, rather than presenting a barrage of criticism. Remain supportive, and show your continued faith in your family member. Mental disorder takes an

enormous toll on self-esteem. Your encouragement and positive attitude – in good times and bad – can erase some of the
damage. *Hope* is a crucial medicine too easily overlooked by
doctors and other professionals.

Remember, the worst of times will surely pass. And when
they do, when things are calm, you can start to plan for the
future. You can set up long-term support systems – medical
and non-medical – so that you know who to call if symptoms
reappear. (Some family members recommend keeping a list of
phone numbers handy – GP, psychiatrist, nearest hospital or
mental health centre.) Together, you can agree on steps to take
next time. For example, the family organization AMI-Quebec
has something called the "Share & Care Telephone Network."
The service puts families in crisis in touch with an experienced "buddy," who offers practical and emotional support
until the crisis passes.

It's also helpful for consumers and family members to learn
the warning signs of relapse – specific behaviours or moods that
become apparent first – and the triggers or stressors that can
induce them. These will vary with each individual, but with time,
you'll come to know them, and how to deal with them early.

A couple of years ago, it seemed that Scott might be becoming unwell again. It was a frightening prospect, until a friend
of ours offered some perspective: "It will never be that bad
again. You have knowledge, and support systems in place now."
She was right.

Remain hopeful and explore external supports

Navigating the System

This is at least as frustrating for family members as it is for
consumers. You can face an awful lot of closed doors. Health
professionals may refuse to meet with you, answer your
questions, or include you in the decision-making process.

Many family members are shocked to find themselves
excluded, but there's a reason for it. Doctors (and other

professionals) have legal and ethical obligations regarding confidentiality. Whether it's a hospital, community service provider, or doctor's office, they can't share specific information – about the diagnosis, treatment plan, their observations, or discussions with their client – unless the consumer explicitly agrees to this.

Most consumers, when asked, will agree to share information. But sometimes professionals don't ask. Doctors vary widely in their regard for family members. Some psychiatrists, for example, will allow family members to attend a session as required; others permit no contact whatsoever. Some feel it's essential to include you; others may regard you with suspicion, even consider you part of the problem rather than the solution.

If your loved one winds up with a service provider who chooses to exclude you, your options are limited. All you can do is provide your own information. If you can't see the professional in person, then do it by telephone or letter. They should always receive your concerns, observations, and requests. (Some family members keep a journal, in which they make note of behaviour changes.) But there are no guarantees these will be taken into account, however valid your input may be.

"He [the doctor] sees her for 15 minutes once a week if I'm lucky," one family member told the "Hear Me Now" study. "I live with her the rest of the time. Now you tell me who is in a better position to decide what should or should not be done for her. I think I am, but the doctors have all the power."

If you feel strongly that you want in on the treatment plan, it's possible to ask your family member to sign a legal document permitting the physician to discuss your case. But only do this if your family member is agreeable. Some consumers, understandably, feel it's a violation of their privacy.

In dealing with professionals, it's best to be pleasant *and* persistent. "If you're just pleasant and you're not persistent, you're not going to get anywhere," says Kitchen, a social worker at a large Toronto hospital. "If you're just persistent without being pleasant, you're going to tend to turn people off."

Telling a doctor how to do his or her job is bound to antagonize. Better to take notes on what you see and hear, and translate that to the doctor. "Let the doctors do their job," says Neasa Martin, "and you do yours, which is giving them the information they need in order for a joint decision to be made."

During a hospital stay, some doctors will agree to (or even initiate) a family meeting. Social workers, occupational therapists, and nurses may also be present. Together, you can discuss treatment options and share information. It's helpful to prepare a list of questions, and points you'd like to raise, in advance. If a meeting isn't offered, feel free to request one.

You can also request meetings with a hospital social worker; they usually work directly with families, and can help you deal with some of your own issues. They can also help with discharge planning, and arrange for home supports if these will help you and your relative. Bear in mind, though, that family members aren't always notified prior to discharge. Some consumers prefer it that way.

For daily updates on your family member's progress, try phoning the assigned nurse: nurses spend more time with a patient than doctors do, and they're more likely to answer your calls. If you need to speak with the doctor, book a time well in advance.

You can help your family member best by knowing the rules and patient rights of the hospital, and by serving as an advocate. Visit often, and bring supplies your loved one may not have packed. (Some professionals recommend frequent *short* visits rather than long ones.)

If your family member has chronic and frequent relapses, he or she can also give you power of attorney (see Chapter 6). This authorizes you to make treatment and/or financial decisions on their behalf, should they become incapable of doing so.

Be patient, polite, and persistent when dealing with the medical system

Supporting Yourself

Remember that old axiom – you have to help yourself to help others? It definitely applies here. And yet with mental disorder it's so easily overlooked. Your loved one's needs and suffering seem so much greater than your own. Your focus is on him or her getting well, not on you *staying* well.

"Time and again, when families are asked what they need . . . they reply in terms of the needs of the ill person only – they don't mention themselves," the *You Are Not Alone* handbook notes. "Many family members do not seem to realize that perhaps we need help too, on our own account, for our own mental and physical health."

On a basic level, helping yourself means eating and sleeping and exercising regularly so that *you* don't become ill, either physically or mentally. And it means maintaining your usual schedule as much as possible: going to work, looking after your kids, attending classes.

It also means making time for yourself, to do things that give you pleasure. Go out with your friends, take a walk, see a movie, buy your favourite magazine and enjoy it in a café. This is especially important in periods of stress, when you're feeling all-consumed by your loved one's disorder.

Taking care of yourself is *not* selfish. Burnout is common and it helps no one. The goal, through this ordeal, is to keep the disorder from taking over, either for your family member or in your own life. As one mother of an adult son with bipolar disorder told us, "If we all get on with our lives, he is much happier."

Looking after yourself also means letting people help you: friends, family, anyone who offers. (This includes your unwell family member!) And if no one offers, then ask. Too often, family members try to manage on their own and end up isolated and depressed.

"I believe that support is essential," says Dr. Geist. "And whether you get the support from the Society or the family or friends, one of the natural antidotes for depression and isolation is getting support that understands."

Many family members report being disappointed with their friends. It seems they can't relate to your pain, or understand the choices you've made. As a spouse, your friends may be surprised you aren't filing for divorce. As a parent, you may feel judged, seen as a bad mother or father who's raised a deviant child. Most family members say some friends (and many neighbours) abandon them. "They feel it's contagious," says Doris Sommer-Rotenberg. "They don't want to be contaminated. They won't have anything to do with you. I was shunned. . . . It's very hard. I fortunately had a few friends who were very devoted, and very understanding."

The hopeful part of that statement comes at the end. Most of us will have at least one friend or relative who *is* supportive. Someone you can call at three in the morning if need be. Make the most of these nurturing relationships; let people be there for you, both as sympathetic listeners and as providers of practical support, whether it's doing the dishes, shopping for groceries, or providing child care.

Self-help groups are also extremely helpful. As we've seen in Chapter 6, you can find them across the country. Many provide workshops, seminars, and information geared to families. They also run regularly scheduled support groups, where family members can share their experiences, their wisdom, and sympathy. People find these groups are a warm sanctuary, and the source of much comfort.

"Probably the first thing is the sense they are not alone," says Ella Amir, executive director of AMI-Quebec, "that they haven't done anything bad to grant this situation."

"In a group, they get education, they get skills, they get emotional support, particularly around the crisis," Dr. Geist says. "They learn how to speak to the doctor, they learn about symptoms of the disease. And they learn from people who they can believe in, because all the families have gone through it."

Counselling is another option. A qualified therapist can help you come to terms with the disorder, and your emotions surrounding it. Grief, guilt, anger, fear, and helplessness are all common feelings that need to be acknowledged.

"Conflicting emotions are normal," Kitchen told a meeting of family members at the Mood Disorders Association in Toronto. "You need to understand and accept them. This helps you remain calm during times of stress, and manage difficult times from within."

At a time when so much attention is focused on your loved one, a therapist can be there for you and you alone, addressing *your* needs, your pain.

"I have no bones about saying that I spent two years in psychotherapy," one family member states, "which has been the best thing I've ever done. Because I needed to grieve all that happened to me. . . . If I hadn't done that, I don't think I'd be as happy as I am. Everyone deserves to have their needs met."

And because everyone's needs, reactions, and rate of adjustment are different, it's important to remember the rest of the family. When one member is unwell, the dynamics of the whole group are bound to change, sometimes in destructive ways. "The blaming and the shame and the stress can produce additional stress, which can debilitate a family," says Dr. Geist. "So they have to learn to work together within the family and not blame each other. And sometimes it's not easy to do that alone."

Some find family counselling helpful – an opportunity to discuss and share how everyone is feeling. Others might prefer to discuss things at home. Either way, it's important to keep the lines of communication open, and allow every family member to be involved in his or her own way.

Children, in particular, need help making sense of what's happened. A CMHA B.C. guide for family members, called *Who Turned Out the Light?*, notes that siblings "often feel grief, anxiety, guilt, lowered self-esteem, self-doubt, preoccupation, jealousy, resentment, stigma, shame, feelings of loss, hopelessness, and a desire to escape." It adds that children living with a parent who has a mental disorder "may be confused and upset with the parent's behaviour. An open discussion with the children regarding the parent's illness may be helpful as well as seeking ongoing support for the children."

In the best of worlds, family members work together as a unit, spelling each other off, drawing on each other's strengths, helping in their own individual ways. Because one person can't do everything.

Admit this to yourself. And when you're feeling especially overwhelmed, don't beat yourself up for being human.

Caregivers need to take care of themselves, too

FOR FRIENDS

Anyone who doubts that friendship makes a difference need only look at the research. It shows that friends can actually affect the course of a disorder. One Canadian study tracked the social and occupational functioning of people with schizophrenia, both eighteen months and five years after their first psychotic episode. It found that people who had strong networks of friends fared better than people who did not. The paper concluded that "greater involvement with and higher quality of social relationships make for better prognosis in schizophrenia." Sadly, the study also found that people with schizophrenia generally had *fewer* friends than people without the disorder, who had also been tracked.

Consumers have told us repeatedly that disorder takes an enormous toll on friendships. We were luckier than most; our strongest friendships endured and were strengthened. A critical core of people stood by us, and if you're reading this book, you probably want to be able to do the same. Here's how.

Give Moral Support

Your friend needs lots of this. Your moral support will help him or her face the many challenges presented by the outside world. Stigma. Rejection. Discrimination. You'd be amazed at all your friend must endure.

"Some people are afraid of you," one consumer says. "They're afraid they're going to get what you have."

True friends, then, are especially important. In fact, some consumers find friends more supportive than family. One woman described what that loyalty meant to her: "It meant that I had a hope of being normal again, the fact that I had two friends who stuck by me."

Moral support means phoning and visiting when your friend is unwell. People often wonder if this is a good idea – Will she want to see me? How will I react to seeing him like that? – but regular contact is an important way to show you care.

"If the friends know you're sick and come to see you anyway, that means a lot," one woman told us. "It means they're your friends even in bad times."

Bear in mind, though, that your unwell friend might push you away, sound abrupt on the phone, refuse to make plans. Don't take this personally. Shame is often part of the landscape of mental disorder; your friend might not want to be seen in a rough state. Withdrawal might also be a symptom; the prospect of even going for coffee can be a daunting task for someone who's depressed. One man told us he "hibernates," avoiding friends when he's depressed. "I think of myself as a likeable fellow that people like to be around. . . . I don't want them to see this other side of me."

In our own case, when Scott was depressed, he often felt obliged to be good company, and was left utterly drained by visits from friends. Even so, we both appreciated the show of support.

So don't retreat or give up on your friend, however unsociable he or she seems. Check in on a regular basis – but with the knowledge that a conversation might not be possible. Even if they don't return phone calls, keep leaving messages that are supportive – just try not to push.

"What works for me," says one understanding friend, "is calling and saying, 'If you're feeling up for it . . .' or, 'When you're ready . . .'"

While you *are* together or talking on the phone, be yourself. Try to understand what your friend is going through. Listen carefully, offer hope, optimism, and encouragement.

"Tell them it definitely will end," one woman stresses. "The first time I was depressed, I thought it would never end. It lasted nine months, but it did end."

If your friend is a family member of someone with a disorder, do all the same things. Family members need moral support too; they're also living with stigma and high stress.

"I guess you could say my need is for people to understand that I am in pain," one family member told the "Hear Me Now" researchers, "that it is as real as tears, and I just need to be allowed to feel it."

Friends can offer just that kind of understanding.

Offer Practical Support

We've already stressed the importance of educating yourself. You can also provide practical support for your friend by providing information – books, pamphlets, useful phone numbers. Both consumers and family members report that they're unsure where to look for this kind of information, and that they lack the time to do so.

In fact, this is one thing few of our friends thought to do. We can think of one exception – it made a big impression, despite the stresses we were under – a friend who called to ask how he could help. We couldn't think of anything concrete, but when he came to visit, he'd done some research. He brought with him a book by William Styron, about the renowned writer's experience with depression. It was a beautifully written story (highly recommended – see the Appendix), which we devoured straight away. And we both took comfort in knowing that Styron had overcome a depression as severe as Scott's.

Resource materials can also help someone accept the need for medical help. One mother whose son has schizophrenia told the CMHA's B.C. Early Intervention Study how his girlfriend went about this task: "She was the first one who even said schizophrenia. She brought literature and a video home, and they sat down and watched it. . . . Watching the video was easier to do with her rather than with his family. . . . Shortly after that, he said he'd be willing to see somebody."

When the disorder is at its most severe, and crisis mode sets in, practical supports become especially important. For consumers and family members, the day-to-day business of life becomes overwhelming. Buying groceries, cleaning the house, paying bills can be major undertakings.

"It's as if you're flat out in bed with the flu," says a social worker. "You can't do things the way you can when you're well. So friends have to take some of that on . . . really practical stuff like bringing over some food or saying, 'Why don't you let me clean your bathroom for you, or walk the dog, or take the kids for the day?'"

When your friend's in hospital, you can bring clothes, slippers, and other comforts from home. "Getting your keys, going to your house, picking up stuff and bringing it back – that shows you care, and it's also very helpful," says Maria, who has been hospitalized more than once.

Offering help ("If there's anything I can do, let me know") is one thing. Asking how to help ("What can I do for you?") is another. These statements show you care, but the most likely response will be "I don't know" or "Thanks anyway." Much better just to step in with something concrete. Like the friend who offered the use of his calling card when we were in crisis in Hong Kong. He urged us to make as many calls home as we liked, without worrying about the expense. It was simple, practical, and incredibly thoughtful, a valuable lifeline at a time when we were completely isolated. Precisely the kind of help we would not have thought to ask for.

Close friends might also succeed where family members have failed in encouraging someone to seek help. At a family member's request or on their own initiative, they can respectfully voice their concern. Ask what your friend thinks is going on. Mention the changes you've noticed, and the reasons for your concern. Do so in a non-threatening, non-judgmental way; sometimes a friend can do this more effectively than a relative.

What's important here is that you be a close and *trusted* friend. And if your suggestion is ignored, painful as it may be, you must be willing to keep offering support. As Doris Sommer-Rotenberg says, it's important "to accept where they are . . . to be able to enlarge our minds to incorporate other people's feelings – as different as they may be from ours."

True friendship is blind to disorder

ON THE JOB

Mental disorder is a multi-billion dollar concern for North American businesses. And it's growing. Data on depression alone confirms this. As much as 20% of an average workforce will show symptoms of depression in a given year, says Bill Wilkerson, president of the Canadian and Economic Roundtable on Mental Health. In a company of 1,000 employees, that's 200 people.

"Of those 200, something like 25 will get detected and diagnosed," he says. "And of those 25, you're going to get 12 who are treated, and 9 who are successfully treated. So the investment opportunity for the company [in guiding employees toward help] is enormous."

As those numbers indicate, there's enormous resistance to seeking help. And when misconceptions about mental disorders taint the workplace, that only adds one more barrier. It's not only hard for the depressed person – it's also costing the corporate world a fortune in lost productivity and potential. A key mission of the roundtable is to show how mental health *is* a business issue. Working with mental health professionals, the roundtable is also trying to dispel some myths.

"Many employers and employees have unwarranted fears and see persons with psychiatric disabilities as unskilled, unproductive, unreliable, violent or unable to handle workplace pressures," reads a Canadian Psychiatric Association (CPA) paper on mental disorders and work. "This stigma creates a climate in which someone who has a problem and needs help may not seek it for fear of being labelled." And when people don't seek help, symptoms can, unfortunately, worsen.

Another problem is that employers or co-workers might not recognize an underlying mental health issue. Rather than look for symptoms, a pamphlet published by the U.S. National Mental Health Association suggests keeping an eye on significant changes in work habits, attendance, behaviours, or performance. Some of the common signals include:

- frequent absences or consistent late arrivals;
- marked and lasting decrease in productivity;
- problems with concentration, decision-making, remembering things;
- increased accidents or safety lapses;
- low morale;
- reduced interest, involvement, or enthusiasm;
- making excuses for poor work or missed deadlines.

Most employees satisfy some of those criteria at one point or another. We all have bad days or weeks, periods when we're having a difficult time. When these start to become a pattern over an extended period of time – and when they're a marked departure from the employee's usual habits – they could be a sign of a mental health problem.

"Quite often you'll notice that someone whose performance has been good, suddenly they're showing less [productivity] than they used to," says Wilkerson.

Suspicions of mental health issues present something of a dilemma for a manager. Implying someone may be suffering from a mental health problem could lead to a lawsuit or union grievance. It could also irreparably damage the relations between the employee and their supervisor. Allowing the performance to continue to slide, however, doesn't accomplish much for either the business or the employee.

Mindful of the moral and legal implications, the roundtable has crafted a strategy for employers or supervisors who may suspect a mental health problem, especially depression. The full guidelines can be found at <http://gpeinternational.com>. Click on "Insights."

Returning to Work

In cases where the employee goes on disability for an extended period, returning to work can be a daunting step.

"Of all persons with disabilities," notes the CPA paper, "those with a mental illness face the highest degree of stigmatization in the workplace."

Many people have told us they were treated very differently upon their return to work. Some felt ignored, shunned. They were also faced with the assumption that a mental disorder somehow negated an entire career's worth of job skills.

In one case, a woman working at a psychiatric teaching hospital found herself effectively demoted after suffering from mood swings. You might expect her employer, fully aware of her diagnosis, to have been sympathetic. But the woman claims this was not so.

Even in mental health agencies, she told us, there is discomfort with psychiatric illnesses and, in particular, with the "concept of having a 'psych patient' as an employee." The woman has taken her case to the Canadian Human Rights Commission.

A receptive and progressive workplace can, by contrast, actually assist in the recovery process. Welcoming someone back, showing you value their contribution (or that you just plain missed them), can do wonders for someone making those first, tentative steps back to work. It takes enormous courage to walk into the workplace after being off for a period of weeks or months. Especially when people know you've been absent for reasons of mental health.

"Recovery from a mental disorder is different, obviously, than recovery from . . . some sort of familiar physical problem," says Wilkerson. "And I think managers and supervisors have to become more appreciative of the recovery process itself: what that means, what it takes."

Depending on the nature of the problem, reasonable accommodation can usually be made for the returning employee – which could be as simple as moving a person with seasonal affective disorder closer to a window. Reduced hours or flex time may be considered for a person uncomfortable with a full shift.

But employers shouldn't let their misunderstanding of mental disorder falsely lower their expectations. Consumers who return to positions of reduced responsibility often express anger or frustration at the turn of events; the new position can serve as a constant reminder that they are now viewed as somehow flawed.

The best results occur when employees feel they can freely and confidentially discuss their disorder with a manager – and when employers educate themselves. In all cases, employees should be treated with the same respect they were accorded prior to the disorder.

"Just because we're crazy," goes a tongue-in-cheek consumer motto, "doesn't mean we're stupid."

An enlightened employer realizes disorders don't negate skills

HEALTHY PRACTICES

There are several small steps consumers can take on that journey towards recovery. Steps that are helpful, but not easy. They can break the monotony of waiting for things to improve, and may even speed recovery. Friends, family members, and colleagues can help by encouraging these practices:

- Exercise. This is a *proven* way to improve mental health – but also one of the hardest things to do, especially when depressed. Even a walk or bike ride will help, particularly in pleasant surroundings. In addition to the physical benefits, it provides a welcome change of scenery, and many consumers say it improves their mood.

- Nutrition. A decent diet can also be a challenge for people who are unwell. Preparing something to eat can seem like a monumental task. And family members sometimes notice that changes in eating habits can worsen symptoms. Proper meals are definitely helpful, even if the person doesn't relish the food.

- Patience. If the person has just been placed on medication or started psychotherapy, be aware that these treatments will take time to work. In this era of medical miracles, it's hard to understand why there are so few quick fixes for mental disorder. The waiting period is frustrating, but it helps if everyone accepts that things *will* get better with time.

- Don't give up. For consumers, friends, and family members alike, this may be the hardest – but most important – strategy of all. As impossible as it may seem, be assured that life is not over. The authors know this from personal experience, and from meeting scores of consumers who have overcome crushing setbacks. *Accept* that recovery will take time, *have faith* things will improve, and take whatever *action* you can to achieve wellness.

NANCY'S STORY *

*Mental illness is in my family. I was lucky; my brother wasn't.
He suffers from schizo-affective disorder. Some want to say he
has a personality disorder too. I reserve judgment on the latter.
If I had to deal with as many hospitalizations – twenty-five in
sixteen years – my personality might be disordered too.*

*My response to his mental illness has changed over time. At
first, I wept. He was an athlete; he played hockey on a Canadian
championship team. Then I got angry. Surely he could "pick up
his socks." Then I was ashamed. Maybe, if I hid out a few thousand miles away, no one would know. Finally, after repeated
contacts with him and the system, I saw that ignorance, fear, and
discrimination were at the root of our society's approach to
mental illness. It was time to get active.*

*Community action also runs in my family. My great-
grandfather was a Presbyterian minister in rural Manitoba in the
1880s. He and my great-grandmother worked to support communities long before there was a Ministry of Health or Human
Resources. My father was a paratrooper in World War II and*

---

* Nancy Hall is British Columbia's Mental Health Advocate, and is quoted in Chapter 6.

later became an Appeal Court judge in the province of Manitoba. My mother was a schoolteacher for pregnant teens in inner-city Winnipeg. Her response to my brother's illness was to advocate for adolescent treatment services. She received an Order of Canada for her volunteer efforts, and I like to think young people with mental illnesses in Manitoba have a somewhat easier time due to her efforts.

There isn't much I can do to change my brother's situation, but he does deserve a better life. As a family member and with twenty years of experience working in the health care field, I have become British Columbia's first Mental Health Advocate. Although my brother's illness doesn't really allow us to be close to one another, in his own way he continues to teach me what counts and what needs doing.

People talk about psychiatric patients' need for medicine in the same breath as diabetics' need for insulin. But it isn't so simple. The meds don't always work, and the side effects are often unpleasant. The science of mental illness is horribly imprecise. For a condition that affects one in five Canadians, it is a national travesty that research into mental illness represents less than 4% of the total Canadian medical research effort.

My brother taught me that meds are but a small part of the picture. The real issue is the constant struggle for dignity that people living with a mental illness experience. As a society, we attach no blame to someone who develops a physical illness, but when it comes to mental illness, people experience discrimination on a daily basis. The community blames the mentally ill for their symptoms and marginalizes them from community life with unfounded fears and prejudice.

There is no reason for a diagnosis to be a sentence to poverty or jail. The reality is that, initially, the illness interferes with a person's ability to work. Forced to live on difficult-to-obtain disability benefits, safe and affordable housing is virtually non-existent.

Seeking care is in many cases a humiliating experience. Most people enter the system in crisis and from then on face a series of hurdles. If they are lucky, they get admitted to hospital; if they are not, they get taken to jail. Approximately one-third of the inmates in B.C. Corrections suffer from a mental disorder. With all the fuss about health-care wait lists, I frequently remind people the mentally ill wait too – only in jail.

My brother taught me it is important to do whatever you can to foster respect and dignity for someone with a mental illness. It is also important to address trauma. Between 50 and 70% of people with a serious mental illness have experienced some form of physical or sexual abuse. Further, many tell me that the care system reactivated that trauma. But few in the care system wish to address trauma.

So what can be done? Like anything, action is progressive and starts from the personal as it moves to the collective. People living with mental illness have many hurtful encounters with their families, their communities, and service systems. As Advocate, I have learned first and foremost to help people self-advocate. To be effective, I have learned that being angry about past injustices is a waste of time. On many occasions, I have found myself asking people, "Do you want to be right, or get well?" People cannot rewrite their past. Caregivers rarely apologize. The only thing a person can do is grieve the past and, when they are ready, create their futures.

Mental illness is so common, if all who were affected stood up and said it isn't good enough we could begin to see the resources required to build the system we need. And keep in mind, there is more to health than health care. Jobs, housing, better access to disability benefits and education are as basic as health care.

I know it's going to be different for my children and their peers. There will no longer be the stigma that we experience today. What's your vision?

CHAPTER EIGHT

"Meds"

"Lithium saved my life" – Pierre

"Lithium robbed my soul" – Joyce

Pierre and Joyce share the same diagnosis – bipolar affective disorder – and little else. Pierre takes his medication daily and credits it with bringing stability to what was a roller-coaster life; Joyce can't stand the way lithium makes her feel and is now trying to manage her disorder without the aid of pharmaceuticals. Both have made an informed decision based on the severity of their disorder and their personal reaction to the medication.

Psychiatric drugs are a two-edged sword. For many Canadians, they're a life-saver. They can provide a much-needed assist to climb out from the depths of depression or escape the crush of a panic attack. They can mute incessant and unwanted voices. They can reduce overwhelming symptoms to the stage where the person is able to benefit from psychotherapy. (Some people are so depressed they are unable to speak. Only after taking an antidepressant are they able to participate in meaningful therapy.)

That's the good news. But there's bad news, too.

Some antipsychotic drugs can cause debilitating, even permanent, side effects. These medications, particularly at higher doses, can leave a person so impaired that they make a conscious choice to stop taking them – even when they are aware of the consequences. Others may find it hard to take medication regularly because it is a constant reminder of their disorder. Conversely, some people with anxiety or sleep disorders can become so dependent on medications that they find it very difficult to cope without them.

It's tough to make a sweeping statement about psychiatric medications, because, as with everything else in the mental health field, the experiences of real people run a very wide gamut. We've met individuals who, after suffering through years of untreated psychosis, are now doing very well on the newest so-called "atypical" medications. We've met others who've developed involuntary facial twitches and grimaces as a direct result of taking antipsychotic drugs. Some folks have emerged from deep depression through therapy and understanding; others have found that it was a pill, not compassion, that saved their life. Many have recovered through combining both.

There can be little doubt that these medications can – and do – work for many people. Most of us will have seen the success stories on magazine covers about Prozac and other "wonder drugs." What's less well-known, however, is the downside of the revolution in psychiatric drugs: the side effects that go hand-in-hand with many of them. Because these side effects have been less publicized, we feel it's important to highlight the most common ones here.

The information that follows should not be interpreted as an endorsement or indictment of any particular medication – and readers currently on a psychiatric medication should not make any changes except under the explicit advice and supervision of their doctor.

INFORMED CONSENT

Regardless of the medication – whether it's for anxiety or blood pressure – you have the right to be fully informed. The prescribing physician has a duty to obtain what's known as your "informed consent." That means they must explain to you the anticipated benefits *and* side effects of the drug prescribed. They must describe the pros and cons of whatever alternative treatments may be available – and the pros and cons of receiving no treatment at all. They must also answer any questions you might have. Only then can you give informed consent.

Unfortunately, consumers commonly complain that they were treated without informed consent. They say they were unaware their medication could cause certain side effects. Even more commonly, they say they were not told about alternative treatments or that they could decline treatment.

There have been a number of lawsuits recently in the United States, many of them successful, in which patients sued their doctors for failing to inform them adequately of these facts. For that reason – and for reasons of good ethical practice – more and more physicians document that they have obtained informed consent and add that material to the patient's records.

However, a study published in the *Canadian Journal of Psychiatry* in 1998 indicated that very few of the psychiatrists surveyed were following this practice. It found that of thirty psychiatrists (each of whom had at least ten patients on antipsychotic medication), documentation of informed consent appeared in only 23% of patients' records. The study also found that while 67% of psychiatrists stated they "always or almost always" told patients about the risk of a serious movement disorder (tardive dyskinesia) caused by some antipsychotic drugs, 27% mentioned this side effect only "sometimes," while 6% mentioned it "never or almost never."

In other words, it's a good idea to insist that your physician describe *all* the benefits and risks of taking any psychiatric medication.

Pharmacists know drugs. And few pharmacists know psychiatric medications better than Kalyna Butler, co-editor of the *Clinical Handbook of Psychotropic Drugs*. Now in its tenth edition, the handbook is regarded by many clinicians as *the* source for information on medications, their side effects, and their interactions with other drugs. Butler, former acting head of Pharmacy for the psychiatry side of the Centre for Addiction and Mental Health, believes it's important for people to be aware of benefits and risks whatever the medication.

"*Any* drug," she emphasizes, "I don't care what it is. Aspirin, for example – people should know the risks. I would want to know, and everybody should know."

A good source of information for the layperson is something called the CPS, the *Compendium of Pharmaceuticals and Specialties*. It lists all drugs currently marketed in Canada, along with their recommended doses, side effects, and interactions. The CPS is available at major bookstores and, quite often, at your local pharmacy. It's a worthwhile purchase, as this chapter will touch on only some of the more common medications and their side effects.

ANTIDEPRESSANTS

Canadians are now taking these at a record rate for depression and anxiety. The number of people in this country receiving prescriptions for antidepressants leapt from 2.72 million in 1993 to 3.75 million in 1998. The value of those prescriptions totalled $320 million in Canada in 1998. That's a lot of pills. A reasonable question would be: how do they work?

"The reality is, we don't know how any antidepressants work," a noted psychiatrist told fellow physicians at a medical conference. "You can say what they *do*, but you can't say how they *work*."

And that, more or less, is how we have come to classify groups of medications: by what they do. But before we start with antidepressants, a word about what they *won't* do.

Medications do not cure mental disorders. They will not solve the problem that might have triggered a depression or been the seed of an anxiety disorder. They will, however, help a person *cope*. Literature has repeatedly shown that your odds of getting well and staying well are best when you combine medication with therapy. On their own, drugs help with symptoms, not solutions.

It's also worth noting that finding the medication that works best for you can sometimes be a process of trial and error. Some people respond well to certain antidepressants; some do not. A physician may switch or "tweak" medications during the course of your treatment in the hope of finding the most suitable combination.

We should also mention that there is a growing number of books out there that raise cautionary flags regarding long-term use of many psychiatric medications and the increasing prescription of these medications to young people. While our goal is neither to encourage nor discourage use of such drugs, we do recommend that you read as much literature as possible. We've included some books reflecting both sides of this debate in our Appendix.

SSRIs

This class of drugs, like all antidepressants, alters the normal flow of chemical neurotransmitters in the central nervous system. Neurotransmitters are the couriers that allow brain cells to communicate with each other. To get a *very* basic idea of how they work, picture the spot in the brain where neurotransmitters communicate between one neuron and the next as a room. At each end of that room are a number of different-shaped doors.

Under normal circumstances, there's a molecular relay race as chemical neurotransmitters are released through one door, whiz through the room, and find the correct door at the other end. When they put their "key" in the door, that's a signal to the neuron on the other side to continue the relay by releasing more neurotransmitters. The *original* neurotransmitter then does one of two things: it either turns around and finds the door back into the original neuron (reuptake), or it gets broken down (metabolized) by an enzyme.

Antidepressants can be thought of as the keys that lock or unlock certain doors. When the doors are locked, specific neurotransmitters are forced to make changes in their travel plans.

"So I always think of a drug as like a key travelling the body to see which keyhole it can fit into," explains Butler. "And if it fits into the keyhole and turns the lock, it works."

SSRI stands for selective serotonin reuptake inhibitor. That means it locks some of the reuptake doors that allow serotonin – a kind of neurotransmitter – to go back to where it started. This increases the amount of serotonin available to act on the receptor, or "keyhole." The SSRIs make up one of the more recently developed classes of antidepressants and are the most commonly prescribed. And while they're most often associated with treatment for depression, SSRIs are now the first drugs doctors try for treating anxiety.

You've likely seen many news stories that describe depression solely as a biochemical imbalance, stating that those with depression have low levels of serotonin. That may be part of the equation, but it's not nearly that simple. Though these medications boost serotonin levels very quickly, it still takes weeks for depressive symptoms to fade. If depression were due solely to serotonin depletion, the symptoms would be gone the same day you started taking the pills. It's also worth noting that some people do not respond to SSRIs at all.

Drugs in the SSRI class include:

- fluoxetine (trade name Prozac)
- fluvoxamine (Luvox)
- paroxetine (Paxil)
- sertraline (Zoloft)
- citalopram (Celexa).

Although they all affect basically the same serotonin neu-rotransmitter, the types of "keys" each carries around on its keychain differ somewhat. Which means other neurotrans-mitters are also affected, causing slightly different side effects for each medication. Overall, however, there are some side effects common to them all. All of these medications *may* cause:

- dry mouth
- sexual disturbances (impotence, inability to orgasm, delayed ejaculation)
- gastrointestinal troubles (nausea, vomiting, heartburn)
- tremor
- drowsiness, sedation
- insomnia
- headache
- night sweats.

The intensity of these side effects varies from individual to individual and with dosage levels. Many people have no problem at all. Some side effects, like dry mouth, can be made more tolerable by sucking on a sour candy or chewing sugar-less gum. People often find side effects lessen during the first couple of weeks as their body adapts to the medication, though that's not always the case. Most people find side effects vastly preferable to the hell of depression.

Typically it takes about a month before a patient feels like the depression is starting to lift. People who are both depressed and lethargic frequently find their energy level gets a boost before their mood does. Paradoxically, this can increase the risk of suicide for a depressed patient who would like to die but lacks the energy to carry out the act. The pharmaceutical literature provided to physicians frequently warns them to keep close tabs on suicidal patients being prescribed these medications.

Most people stay on antidepressants for several months or longer, until their depressive symptoms have fully lifted and they've returned to a stable mood. For many Canadians, that's it. The physician may then recommend a slow tapering off from the drug, since many people encounter side effects (dizziness, nausea, overactive dreams) if they stop the medication abruptly. People with a history of depressive episodes will frequently be kept on the drug "prophylactically" on a long-term basis to prevent depression from recurring.

SSRIs, along with other antidepressants, have been known to trigger hypomania or mania in some people, so it's important to let your physician know of any family history of bipolar disorder or any abnormal mood changes you experience. If you start feeling significantly better than your normal, non-depressed self, see your doctor. Kalyna Butler says the risk of this increases if you have a close relative with the disorder. "If there's a history of bipolar disorder in the family," she says, "the risk is much higher – up to 30% or so. If there's no history, then it's less than 10%."

For those people previously diagnosed with bipolar affective disorder who are now in a depression, psychiatrists often prescribe an antidepressant in conjunction with a mood stabilizer. The stabilizer prevents the drug from sending the person soaring into a hypomanic or manic phase. Because there can still be an associated risk, some physicians choose an antidepressant with a short "half-life" – meaning it doesn't take too long to disappear from the body once you stop taking the pills. (Prozac has a relatively long half-life and would be an unlikely first choice for this reason.)

As mentioned, antidepressants have also recently become the first line of treatment for anxiety disorders. They can block the symptoms of panic, including rapid heartbeat, chest pains, and breathing problems – and they do not have the highly addictive qualities of some medications traditionally prescribed for these disorders.

At least one of these medications, however, may have a dark side. A *Boston Globe* article in July 2000 stated that pharmaceutical giant Eli Lilly "has known for years that its best-selling drug [Prozac] could cause suicidal reactions in a small but significant number of patients." Those reactions have allegedly been caused by the drug's potential to cause extreme agitation in some people.

More extensive side-effect profiles for each specific drug can be found in the CPS – or ask your pharmacist. If the medication causes you unmanageable side effects, talk to your doctor.

Other "RIs"

Serotonin is just one of many neurotransmitters dancing around up there. Norepinephrine is another. A class of drugs called selective serotonin norepinephrine reuptake inhibitors (SNRIs) act primarily on those two neurotransmitters, though they also exert a lesser effect on another one called dopamine. One of the more commonly prescribed SNRIs in Canada is venlafaxine, sold under the trade name Effexor. It has many of the same side effects as the SSRI group, though the manufacturer says it has been clinically proven to be more effective than its main competitor. (Drug manufacturers love to make claims like that.) SNRIs can cause sweating and elevate blood pressure, with both of these side effects mounting as the dose increases.

SDRIs are selective dopamine reuptake inhibitors. A Canadian example is Wellbutrin. In the competitive world of pharmaceutical marketing, its manufacturer emphasizes the important side effect Wellbutrin does *not* have: sexual dysfunction. A minority of people in clinical trials reported headaches, constipation, dry mouth, nausea, dizziness, and tremor. Again, these side effects can fade or become more tolerable over time. Interestingly, the identical medication is also marketed under the name Zyban as an aid to quit smoking. (You'll notice warnings on their television ads that Zyban should not be taken with an antidepressant. That's because it *is* one.)

Nefazodone (trade name Serzone) is another antidepressant that plays up the sexual angle. Not only will Serzone let you have sex, it'll put you to sleep afterwards. Side effects of this medication can include dry mouth, nausea, dizziness, and sleepiness.

Tricyclics

Tricyclic antidepressants – which get their name from their three-ringed molecular structure – were one of the first classes of drugs developed to treat depression. They too work by increasing the level of key neurotransmitters in the brain, but are not as "selective" as the drugs mentioned above. Though used primarily for depression, tricyclics are also prescribed for panic disorder, narcolepsy, migraine headache, and obsessive-compulsive disorder. Side effects in this class can include sedation, blurred vision, dry mouth, weight gain, muscle twitches, urinary retention or constipation, weakness, and decreased blood pressure.

An overdose of tricyclics poses a greater health risk than most other antidepressants. Symptoms of overdose show up quickly as rapid heartbeat, dilated pupils, and a flushed face. They can quickly become more serious, progressing to confusion, seizures, loss of consciousness, irregular heartbeat, cardiorespiratory collapse, and ultimately death.

Tricyclics prescribed in Canada include:

- amitriptyline (e.g., trade name Elavil, Novo-Triptyn)
- clomipramine (e.g., Anafranil, Novo-Clopamine)
- desipramine (e.g., Pertofrane, Norpramin, PMS-Desipramine)
- doxepin (e.g., Sinequan, Triadapin, Apo-Doxepin)
- imipramine (e.g., Tofranil, Novo-Pramine, Apo-Imipramine)
- nortriptyline (e.g., Aventyl, Norventyl, Apo-Nortriptyline)
- protriptyline (e.g., Triptil)
- trimipramine (e.g., Rhotrimine, Surmontil, Apo-Trimip).

Other cyclic antidepressants include:

- Amoxapine (e.g., Asendin)
- Maprotiline (e.g., Ludiomil).

Another side effect common to the tricyclics is known as "orthostatic hypotension." This basically means that when a person stands up or rapidly changes their position they can get dizzy or faint because of a drop in blood pressure. (Most people find they can adapt to this simply by being cautious and moving a tad more slowly.) Because tricyclics can cause an irregular or rapid heartbeat, it's important to remind your doctor of any history of heart trouble. With certain heart conditions, use of tricyclic medications can be dangerous.

MAOIs

Monoamine oxidase inhibitors also increase neurotransmitter levels – but they have a different way of doing it. Instead of locking doors, MAOIs go after specific enzymes in the brain. Under normal circumstances, these enzymes break down certain neurotransmitters. When MAOIs get in the way, the enzymes can't do that job. As a result, the level of certain neurotransmitters rises. Same ball game, different rules.

But those rules have some implications, because certain enzymes that are "deactivated" are ones that normally break down chemicals found in many common foods. If you eat enough of those foods while on an MAOI, it can trigger a dramatic rise in blood pressure. Your doctor or pharmacist can provide you with a full list of what to cut out of your diet or consume only in moderation. MAOIs prescribed in Canada include phenelzine sulfate (Nardil) and tranylcypromine sulfate (Parnate). Although moclobemide (Manerix) falls under the MAOI category, you don't have to change your diet while taking it.

Because of the way in which MAOIs operate, a person taking these drugs cannot be rapidly switched to a different antidepressant. You must first go through what's known as a "washout" period to ensure there's no residual action before the other drug is started. Taking an MAOI at the same time as another antidepressant must be *strictly* avoided or your serotonin levels can go through the roof. If you're on an MAOI and switch physicians, make sure they know you've been taking the drug.

ANTI-ANXIETY DRUGS

Though certain antidepressants are now the most popular drugs for anxiety disorders, the traditional choice has been to prescribe from a class of drugs known as benzodiazepines. Most people know these as "tranquillizers" – though that's something of a misnomer and these drugs are now commonly called anti-anxiety medications or anxiolytics.

No matter what you call them, benzodiazepines are a fast-acting type of drug that can quell the symptoms of panic and anxiety. Some of them have sedative properties and are also prescribed for sleep disorders. Unfortunately, many people who've been on these medications a while find they can become quite dependent on them. Though psychiatric literature cautions against their use with people who are "addiction-prone," there are many Canadians out there who would argue that benzodiazepines *made* them addicts. A Canadian book called *Out of Tune* critically examines the issue of benzodiazepines and dependence. Its author, Joan Gadsby, took prescription tranquillizers and sleeping pills for twenty-three years and almost died through an accidental overdose.

There are many other Canadians, however, for whom short-term use of benzodiazepines has been very beneficial. The key here is short-term, because some people with anxiety disorders find their symptoms rebound with even greater intensity if they stop taking the drug after longer-term use. Most literature recommends that benzodiazepines be used for a period of only four to six weeks, though there are exceptions.

Withdrawal from benzodiazepines usually involves tapering off slowly under the supervision of a doctor. Abrupt withdrawal after long-term use can trigger very severe side effects, including seizures.

Benzodiazepines prescribed in Canada include:

Short-acting:

- triazolam (e.g., Halcion, Apo-Triazo).

Intermediate:

- alprazolam (e.g., Xanax, Apo-Alpraz, Novo-Alprazol)
- bromazepam (e.g., Lectopam)
- lorazepam (e.g., Ativan, Nu-Loraz)
- oxazepam (e.g., Serax, Novoxapam)
- temazepam (e.g., Restoril).

Long-acting:

- chlordiazepoxide (e.g., Librium, Novo-Poxide)
- clonazepam (e.g., Rivotril, Apo-Clonazepam)
- clorazepate (e.g., Tranxene)
- diazepam (e.g., Valium, Novo-Dipam)
- flurazepam (e.g., Dalmane)
- nitrazepam (e.g., Mogadon, Nitrazadon).

Because benzodiazepines work by suppressing the central nervous system, there are some side effects common to them all: drowsiness, fatigue, dizziness, lack of coordination. Anxiolytics lower the tolerance to alcohol, so drinking and popping a pill is not recommended. If you've been on a benzodiazepine for a long period and want to stop taking the drug, consult your doctor. Do not abruptly discontinue use without medical advice.

In Canada, buspirone (BuSpar) is another common anxiolytic – though it is not classed as a benzodiazepine.

MOOD STABILIZERS

Mood stabilizers, though sometimes used with other disorders, are primarily prescribed in the psychiatric field for bipolar affective disorder. And while they are often used in conjunction with an antipsychotic (see pages 228–35) to bring a person down from an acute manic phase, their most common use is to maintain a stable mood. That means acting to *prevent* both mania and depression.

Lithium, a naturally occurring salt, is likely the best-known mood stabilizer and was, until recent years, the most commonly prescribed. Many Canadians tolerate this medication well and credit it with bringing stability to what was previously a life of unmanageable ups and downs.

For lithium to work effectively, it must reach concentrations in the body that fall within what's known as the therapeutic range. Blood tests will ensure that the concentration is not too weak, rendering the drug ineffective, or too strong, where it can become toxic. Because the rate at which people metabolize lithium can change over time, levels should be checked regularly.

On rare occasions, physicians have been somewhat neglectful in this. Two people we spoke to during our research wound up requiring a kidney transplant because their physicians failed to monitor lithium levels regularly. It's a very extreme and uncommon reaction, however, and one that can be safely avoided with a schedule of blood tests.

Although side effects can include nausea, vomiting, and abdominal pain, these often diminish over time. The most common complaint we heard from users was that lithium left them feeling "flat." Some suggested that it interfered with their creativity – though others felt side effects were a small price to pay for stability. Adverse reactions can also include weight gain and slight tremors or shakiness, especially in the hands.

People taking lithium should be aware that anything which lowers the level of sodium in their body can cause lithium levels to rise. If you start a low-salt diet, or begin an exercise program where you're sweating heavily, or have a major bout of diarrhea or vomiting, let your doctor know; it may be necessary to alter your dose.

Precisely why lithium helps to prevent mood swings is unknown. But when people with a diagnosis of bipolar affective disorder abruptly discontinue the drug, roughly half of them experience either a depressive or manic phase within the next three to five months.

The most commonly prescribed mood stabilizer these days, the first-line choice, is divalproex sodium (Epival) or its partner, valproic acid (e.g., Depakene). These anticonvulsants, often used to treat epilepsy, also prevent mood swings. Adverse side effects may include headaches, double vision, anxiety, confusion, dizziness, and weight gain (especially for women). Some women also report menstrual disturbances, and up to 12% of both sexes can experience some degree of hair loss. There have been rare reports of liver dysfunction, so most physicians will order tests, particularly during the first six months on the drug.

Carbamazepine (Tegretol) is another anticonvulsant frequently prescribed for bipolar affective disorder. Though it's not as tricky as lithium to establish and maintain the right level, carbamazepine can affect the blood levels of other medications being taken at the same time. This drug can also occasionally cause a drop in the white blood cell count. For that reason, blood tests are carried out from time to time. That's also why it's important to notify your doctor if you develop a fever, sore throat, or experience unusual bruising while on the drug. The medication can cause skin rashes in up to 15% of people.

Clonazepam (Rivotril) is occasionally prescribed for this disorder, both as a mood stabilizer and as an extra tool in bringing someone down from acute mania. There have been some reports that it is useful for rapid cyclers, people who rapidly alternate between depression and mania. As this drug is a member of the benzodiazepine family, the same side effects and precautions noted earlier apply.

During a depressive phase, it's not uncommon for a physician to combine one of the above mood stabilizers with an antidepressant. Though it may be tempting, a person with a diagnosis of bipolar disorder and who has suffered a previous manic episode should never take antidepressants without mood stabilizers during a depressive phase.

ANTIPSYCHOTICS, OLD AND NEW

These are the big guns in the world of psychiatric drugs. They are used to treat a person in an acute psychotic state and – with schizophrenia in particular – to prevent a return to that state.

They are also used to treat people in hypomanic or manic phases of bipolar affective disorder, and in other instances where psychotic features are apparent.

The experiences of people on antipsychotic medication vary widely. Some find the side effects extremely difficult to tolerate; others find they can function quite well (including work) on appropriate doses of the right medication. It seems to depend largely on dosage, individual metabolism, and the nature and severity of the problem being treated.

What's known as "compliance" – sticking to a medication regimen – is often a problem with antipsychotics. Frequently, this is blamed solely on the consumer's "lack of insight." This term implies that the disorder itself blinds them to their need for medication.

This can be true especially when a person is stable following a first psychotic episode. But we've also seen many people who have made a conscious, informed decision to stop or decrease their medication because, quite simply, to them the treatment feels unbearable. In cases where this is an issue, we recommend that loved ones discuss unpleasant side effects with the person taking the medication and – with the co-operation of a physician – take any possible steps to improve the situation. There may well be options that result in better quality of life for the consumer – including trying a different medication or changing the current dose.

"We do know patients stop their meds because of side effects," says pharmacist Kalyna Butler. "Anybody would. If you were given an antibiotic and had persistent diarrhea, you would probably want to stop it.

"But it's important," she cautions, "to discuss this problem with your doctor first."

Now, a quick overview of antipsychotic drugs.

The first one, chlorpromazine (Largactil), was introduced in the 1950s. It helped dampen the voices associated with schizophrenia and quell psychosis. Its development paved the way for people with severe mental disorders to leave the asylums and live in the community (though many would argue that boarding houses and group homes are, like asylums, just another kind of institution). Since then, a large number of antipsychotic drugs have been developed.

Broadly speaking, these medications are subdivided into drugs known as "typical" or "conventional" agents (e.g., haloperidol, fluphenazine, perphenazine) and "atypical" or "novel" agents (e.g., risperidone, olanzapine).

To a greater or lesser degree, all of these drugs block the neurotransmitter called dopamine. Some attempt to do so fairly selectively (just like the antidepressants that focus on serotonin); others throw up roadblocks to many different neurotransmitters. The selective drugs are referred to in the business as "clean," while the less discriminating ones are often called "dirty."

To a certain extent, side effects can be predicted depending on which neurotransmitters are affected. In other words, on paper at least, the more "clean" the drug is, the fewer the adverse effects. But it doesn't always work out that way. Some "dirty" drugs have relatively few adverse effects – and some clean ones sure don't feel like it. Individual biochemistry plays an important role here; a medication that one person tolerates well can make someone else feel awful. Your body size, metabolism, and even ethnic background can all play a role. (Research has shown that Asians tend to require lower dosages.) Dosages, duration of dose, interaction with other drugs – even diet and smoking – can all affect how an antipsychotic makes you feel.

The "Typicals"

These antipsychotic medications can be taken in a variety of ways. Some are taken orally in tablet or liquid form, some can be mixed with sesame oil and given as a long-acting injection, sometimes called "depot." Antipsychotics like chlorpromazine (Largactil) are relatively low-potency and generally require higher doses; drugs like haloperidol (Haldol) are much more powerful, and less medication is required. Even so, someone who metabolizes Haldol very quickly could require a much higher dose than another person who displays identical clinical symptoms.

The most common side effects of these "typical" or "conventional" antipsychotics are muscular. During initial phases of treatment there can be a reaction called acute dystonia. This involves involuntary muscle spasms, particularly in the trunk, neck, or eyes (the patients' eyes can roll upward). It most often occurs when people have been given fairly heavy doses of antipsychotics to dampen psychosis – a practice known as rapid neuroleptization. A September 1998 supplement to the *Canadian Journal of Psychiatry* described the case of a young man for whom the treatment only reaffirmed his belief that hospital staff were out to harm him.

"Rapid neuroleptization," states the article, "is, unfortunately, a procedure still frequently followed in acute-care hospital situations. In an acute crisis in a busy emergency ward, explanation of undesirable side effects of psychotropic medications is often difficult."

Acute dystonia can be treated with other medication.

"Typical" antipsychotics can also cause restlessness, stiffness, shakiness, and an overall slowing of movement. Some of these effects are referred to as Parkinsonism, as they mimic the symptoms of Parkinson's disease. Again, there are medications that can help ease these side effects.

The restlessness referred to above is clinically termed akathisia. You feel like you can't relax, that you are compelled to shift position. This constant motion is occasionally misinterpreted by physicians as a psychotic symptom, which can lead to the following vicious circle, described in a separate article in the same psychiatry supplement.

"Akathisia, which may occur in 20% to 25% of all patients on antipsychotics, must be differentiated from psychotic agitation to avoid the all too common clinical error of increasing the antipsychotic dose for agitation, which only exacerbates the akathisia."

Other common reactions to "typical" antipsychotics include constipation, drowsiness, dry mouth, sensitivity to the sun, blurred vision, and ejaculatory or menstrual disturbances. There are others, too, but that's quite a handful already. One interesting study in British Columbia found that patients cited side effects as the most common reason (35%) for discontinuing medication.

Perhaps the most troubling potential side effect is known as tardive dyskinesia. It's a condition that develops over time, affects women more than men, affects older people more than younger, and – in some folks – can be permanent. In essence, it produces uncontrollable, involuntary grimacing and twitching in the facial area. A person with a case of TD might smack their lips repeatedly, stick their tongue out, contort their face.

The symptoms can be so pronounced they reinforce our stereotypical view of what "crazy" looks like. Yet they are a result of the treatment, not the disorder. Studies indicate that the longer a person is on antipsychotic medication, the greater their chances of developing the condition.

"What they've found is the first five years are the critical years," says Kalyna Butler. "And 5% of the individuals on a 'typical' antipsychotic will get tardive dyskinesia every year they're on it. So by five years, 25% of the population will have it. The next five-year course is varied. Most get better, some stay the same, and in a small percentage it gets worse."

And yet, according to data released at the 1999 Ontario Psychiatric Association conference, tardive dyskinesia is a side effect a number of doctors avoid mentioning to their patients. They'll explain other common adverse reactions like muscle rigidity, but sometimes fail to warn people about arguably the most severe side effect.

"What tends to happen," explained one of the study's authors, "is that psychiatrists and family physicians tended to inform patients more about the immediate [muscular side effects]. Their rates for disclosure about tardive dyskinesia and neuroleptic malignant syndrome – very few people in Ontario are disclosing."

As the name suggests, neuroleptic malignant syndrome is also caused by antipsychotic drugs. It is very rare – but if undiagnosed it can lead to death. The symptoms are very much like a bad case of the flu and can come on without warning.

"The person gets very rigid, stiff, the blood pressure goes up, the temperature goes up," explains Butler. "They look like they have the flu with severe muscle rigidity. It could be you're on the drug for ten years and suddenly it happens. So there's some trigger they haven't identified."

Butler emphasizes that neuroleptic malignant syndrome is extremely rare. Caught early, it can be treated successfully. (The mortality rate has dropped dramatically during the past twenty years due to greater awareness of the syndrome and earlier intervention.)

The "Atypicals"

The past decade has brought a wave of new "atypical" or "novel" antipsychotic medications. These drugs are at least as effective as the old antipsychotics and have fewer of the negative side effects. For many people with a diagnosis of schizophrenia in particular, these medications have meant a tremendous improvement in quality of life. These next-generation antipsychotics have also been found to control symptoms in many instances where older meds have failed.

Atypicals currently on the market in Canada include:

- clozapine (Clozaril)
- olanzapine (Zyprexa)
- risperidone (Risperdal)
- quetiapine (Seroquel).

When compared with such traditional antipsychotics as haloperidol (Haldol), the atypicals produce fewer muscular side effects. It should be noted, however, that in some of the studies the doses of Haldol given were a lot higher than what is now regarded as standard. In other words, the subjects receiving Haldol may have been experiencing greater side effects than necessary. There's currently strong evidence that, assuming the person does not metabolize Haldol at an irregular rate, symptoms can be controlled in many people with doses ranging from 2 to 10 milligrams per day. Anything beyond that, with most people, is of questionable clinical benefit – and will most certainly increase side effects.

The atypicals have other things going for them. Some studies indicate these novel antipsychotics can reduce the "negative" symptoms of schizophrenia – meaning some of the emotional flatness associated with the disorder. One man with a diagnosis of schizophrenia told us that, after switching to olanzapine, people noticed the difference.

"People treat me more as a human, because now they see a human," he said. "Whereas before they used to see just a blank expression on my face, along with slow movements."

You may hear concerns that olanzapine can cause something called agranulocytosis. This is a severe drop in the number of white blood cells, a reaction that has caused a number of deaths in the United States. Since those deaths, anyone on this drug has their blood checked regularly, and the rate of agranulocytosis is now less than one per cent and fatalities are very rare.

Weight gain can be a significant deterrent with some atypicals, particularly with clozapine and olanzapine. One psychiatrist described seeing patients gain "horrendous" amounts on the latter medication. Some people find that clozapine can cause excessive salivation. Headache, sleepiness, and dizziness have been reported with quetiapine.

Because these medications are relatively new to the market, fewer long-term studies have been carried out to determine their pros and cons. As this book was being prepared for publication, studies were appearing in academic journals indicating that atypicals, though an improvement, are far from perfect. As always, we'd urge people considering taking any medication to investigate thoroughly both its benefits and risks.

It should also be noted, however, that some of the atypicals have allowed people who've been institutionalized for years – and for whom older medications have failed – to return to life in the community. This new class of antipsychotics has spurred much research, so expect further developments in the years to come.

THE GOOD NEWS

You may well think by now that the authors are essentially "anti-antipsychotic." Not so. These medications are improving all the time, and clearly allow tens of thousands of Canadians to live without the ravages of psychosis – allow many, in fact, to hold down a job or return to school. We've met many people for whom neuroleptics do not pose debilitating side effects.

We do, however, have great empathy with those who find their treatment a chemical straitjacket. In their cases, we strongly believe every effort should be made to ensure – whenever possible – that antipsychotics are being used at the *minimum dose* required to obtain therapeutic effects.

There's been a lot of very good science in recent years indicating that people have, traditionally, been given doses of these medications well above what's needed to control their symptoms. There's growing consensus that side effects that were until recently considered a necessary evil are now unacceptable. Unfortunately, not everyone has changed their practice to keep up with the times.

"There are some horrendous doses out there," says Kalyna Butler. In fact, when Butler was at the Centre for Addiction and Mental Health, it wasn't uncommon for family members to call and ask if there was anything that could be done. "We always tell them, 'Discuss this with your doctor first'," she says. "You can, however, get a second opinion if your physician isn't listening."

Scott once received a call from a father concerned for his son. The young man was on high doses of Haldol and was finding it difficult to function. Scott urged the family to contact another doctor. The father later called back. "They've cut the dose in half and he's doing much better," he said. "The doctor thinks they can cut it in half again." Assuming the young man's symptoms remain controlled, he is now on *one-quarter* the dose he was originally prescribed.

Butler stresses that anyone who finds their side effects unmanageable should speak up or seek the opinion of another professional. It's advice she frequently gives to in-patients.

"If you have a troublesome side effect," she tells them, "it is up to you to speak up about it and ask what can be done about it. And if your doctor says 'I can't do anything' – then ask for a second opinion.

"I personally don't believe anybody should have a side effect that's incapacitating to their functioning. Minor ones we all can tolerate, dry mouth or whatever. But not something that's dysfunctional."

Psychiatric drugs, for many, have been the means to achieve a vastly more manageable life. However, it's always worth remembering:

- incapacitating side effects are no longer considered acceptable;
- you have a right to speak up about side effects – and a right to be heard;
- physicians must explain all potential benefits and risks of planned treatment, including the pros and cons of alternative treatments – and the option of no treatment at all;
- you have the right to ask questions;
- you have the right to get answers.

The same rights apply to these final two forms of treatment. Like medications, they take a biological approach, directly targetting the brain. Both are highly controversial, some would say drastic, measures. So if you're considering either of them, it's crucial that you be well-informed about the risks. And that should involve some homework beyond what you'll read here.

ELECTROCONVULSIVE THERAPY (ECT)

We know of no common procedure in the mental health world as controversial as that of passing an electric current through the brain for the purpose of inducing a seizure. We've spoken to practitioners who say they've witnessed miracles with ECT; we've heard from survivors who say they've suffered permanent and extensive memory loss. We've also heard from folks who say it worked for them when nothing else did.

And we believe all of those statements are true.

The notion of using an electrical stimulus to induce a seizure developed in Italy in the late 1930s. When a patient with hallucinations was apparently helped by the procedure, it became more popular – first as a treatment for schizophrenia, then for severe depression and mania.

For decades, however, people receiving ECT did not receive general anaesthetic or muscle relaxants. The accompanying convulsions often caused serious complications for up to 40% of recipients. Compression fractures of the vertebrae were common. ECT declined rapidly in use, and was even banned in some U.S. states.

Since the mid-1980s, however, it's experienced a resurgence. These days, both a muscle relaxant and general anaesthetic are used. Electrodes are applied either to one (unilateral) or both (bilateral) sides of the head. An electrical current is then applied, triggering a seizure in the brain that lasts about one minute. Typically, people will receive six to twelve treatments over a course of several weeks. There's no agreement on the precise "mechanism of action" that takes place in the brain.

ECT is usually recommended for either severe, suicidal depression or for extreme mania – and often only after other medications have failed. It is also used, though not as frequently, with schizophrenia. Critics note that older women seem to receive this treatment in unusually high numbers, and suggest it's being used simply to get people out of hospital as quickly as possible.

ECT always causes some memory loss – usually for the period right around the treatment. Some people, though physicians insist such cases are very rare, say the procedure has cost them much more. You'll hear the stories of two people who had very different experiences with ECT right after this chapter.

The Canadian Psychiatric Association has reviewed the literature and issued a position paper on ECT. It states that, "when used properly, ECT is a safe and effective treatment which should continue to be available as a therapeutic option for the treatment of mental disorders."

We urge you to research this topic extensively before making a decision. One of the more thorough reports we've read manages to balance both scientific data with people's real-life experiences. You can find it at <www.healthyplace.com/Communities/Depression/ect/studies/UKreport.html>.

PSYCHOSURGERY

The practice of operating on the brain for psychiatric reasons has been out of favour for several decades. And for good reason. The lobotomy, performed on tens of thousands of psychiatric patients in the 1940s and 50s, has gone down in history as one of modern medicine's most barbaric practices. The side effects were both common and irreversible: personality changes, impaired judgment and reasoning, seizures, even death.

Today, psychosurgery can still be practised – with a patient's consent – in some U.S. states and Canadian provinces, including Alberta and Ontario. But its use is extremely rare, and limited to people with severe, chronic, and treatment-resistant disorders. (One neurosurgeon in Edmonton told us that in twenty-five years of practice, only three patients had been referred to him for psychosurgery.) Proponents argue that surgical procedures have been improved and refined since the days of the lobotomy; opponents still find the very notion of psychosurgery offensive.

The procedure most often used – although it's still quite rare – is called a cingulotomy. Two small lesions are burned into a part of the brain called the cingulate gyrus, which is thought to play a role in emotional responses. Cingulotomies are used mainly for chronic and otherwise untreatable obsessive-compulsive disorder; one study of eighteen such patients found five responded well and three partially, with "few serious adverse effects" overall. This study, published in 1995 and conducted at Massachusetts General Hospital, where cingulotomies are most often performed, concluded with a comment that's worth emphasizing in regard to any form of psychosurgery: "Cingulotomy remains a last resort treatment for severely incapacitated patients who have not responded to all other state-of-the-art pharmacological and behavioral treatments for OCD and is not to be taken lightly."

WAYNE'S STORY

I spent twenty-five years in a state of confusion and despair.

It started when my brother died and I turned to alcohol. Before I knew it, I was told I was mentally ill and was in and out of psychiatric hospitals. Although the root cause of my problems was my brother's death and my drinking, I had some 108 hospital admissions and approximately eighty electroconvulsive therapy (ECT) treatments from 1967 to 1992. My charts show that I was diagnosed with numerous different illnesses, including schizophrenia. What should have been treatment for an addiction involved ECT treatments and psychiatric medication. The doctors kept giving me more and more medication (every drug under the sun), up to seventeen different pills per day.

As a result of my shock treatments, I am missing large portions of my memory and suffer from chronic severe back pain because I didn't receive enough muscle relaxants during the ECT. My children suffered from the effects of the loss of a parent. My friends didn't know how to respond to my behaviour, the hallucinations and delusions. I did request shock treatments, because maybe I found temporary relief. They would shock me, get me all medicated up, and send me home where I would drive taxi.

Finally, after twenty-five years of this hell, I ended up in a bad car crash. I was charged and convicted with impaired driving. It was the best thing that could have happened to me. It was the beginning of the end. I stopped taking all the meds, refused any more shock, and then a year later quit drinking. I have not been in hospital since, except to visit. Even today, when I walk down the halls of the Lakehead Psychiatric Hospital, patients come up to me and say hi. They know me, but I have no idea who they are. They don't even look familiar. They say I spent a lot of time with them, but I have no memory. Part of me is missing forever.

During my years in the mental health system, some of the professionals recommended that I be taken off all the drugs, given no more shock, and receive proper counselling. My GP chose to ignore this advice without even informing me of their recommendations. This is unacceptable.

Why do we give the doctors this power? Why is it that medical doctors, who are no experts on mental health, can prescribe any psychotropic agents, even against a psychiatrist's advice? Why aren't they required to learn more about mental illnesses before they go around diagnosing and drugging us? I am not saying that there aren't competent professionals, or that you shouldn't listen to your doctor. What I am saying is that you should make sure you are making an informed decision, and ensure that the communication is there between your psychiatrist and GP.

What has personally helped me is the counselling and peer support I receive from a self-help group I am actively involved with. I am dead set against ECT under any circumstances. Why should delivering electricity through the brain be anything less than destructive and damaging?

D A V I D ' S   S T O R Y *

I'm sixty-six years old. I had severe depression. My wife died in 1991, and by 1994 I was at a point where I had more debts than

---

* "David" is a pseudonym. His words were taken from the transcript of an interview with the authors.

I could cover. So I sat down with pencil and paper one day and figured it out, and boy did I feel depressed. It just kept getting worse from there on.

I was suicidal at the time, and I've still got a few scars on my wrist. Fortunately, at that time in my life I'd sold all my guns; I used to have a handgun and three rifles. I'm quite sure that if I'd been in possession of them I could have cheerfully blown my head off.

I made several attempts on my life. I was going to jump off a bridge one day, but I carelessly let this information slip and my girlfriend stopped me. I did the standard razor-blade routine, but missed the artery. I tried leaving the car running in the garage, but I just got sick. I was hospitalized after some of these attempts. I felt like I would be spending the rest of my life in a revolving door. It was bad.

I was on various drugs and seeing a psychiatrist. My house where I'd lived for twenty-three years was being sold from under me. I stayed with my daughter, and she came home one day to find me facing the wall with all the lights out. She took me straight to the hospital, where I spent about two months. That's where I had the ECT, in the fall of 1994.

The doctor went over all the bad news about it, how the technique had been refined, about the anti-convulsants and the relaxants. I also talked to Helen Hutchison (a former television journalist who herself had ECT). I looked at her very carefully as I talked to her, listening for coherence, and she seemed perfectly coherent. So I decided to give it a try. I was also at the point where I just didn't give a damn if there were any memory effects. I'd have willingly tried anything. I don't know if it was the last hope or not; I was just in pain and I wanted out, in a positive sense.

Afterwards, I didn't feel any different. The first thing I thought of was that I'd heard so much about memory, and I thought, What was my late grandmother's phone number? I recalled that phone number. I also tried to remember the birthdays of my children, and I tried to remember what was going on on the hospital floor. My recall seemed to be quite good.

By the second session, the treatment really broke through for me. Have you ever been in an airplane on the tarmac on a rainy day and the airplane takes off and suddenly you break through the clouds? Well, that was what ECT did to me. It was like breaking through the clouds. I was absolutely astounded at what had happened to me. Bang, I was through the clouds and it felt good. I haven't been back to hospital since January of 1995.

If someone's been in a prolonged period of depression, if medications are not working for them, I think they should seriously consider it. It made a difference for me.

CHAPTER NINE

The Alternatives

Twenty years ago, William Boyd was earning big bucks as a senior manager in the banking industry in Edmonton. Working seven days a week, twelve hours a day, he started to burn out. When the bank transferred him to Toronto, things went from bad to worse. Everything he owned was burned in a moving truck. He was unhappy in his new position. And it started to show.

"I was a basket case," he recalls. "I couldn't handle the anxiety."

Eventually, he resigned. Doctors diagnosed him with bipolar disorder and put him on medication. It didn't help. He was severely depressed. For three years he stayed in his room, venturing downstairs only to eat. His savings drained away; he wound up living on a disability allowance.

"I was seeing a psychiatrist and he wasn't helping me," Boyd says. "I had been an intelligent, productive person, and all he was doing was keeping me like a vegetable. . . . If I'd stayed on the medication, I'd still be a zombie."

So Boyd tried something different, something a growing number of North Americans are now using for all kinds of ailments. He went to a practitioner of alternative medicine and replaced the meds with a carefully crafted regime of vitamins and herbs. With his wife, he started researching – and practising – spirituality and healthy living. "All during the fourteen years since I quit the bank, I've been a voracious reader, all non-fiction, all about health and spirituality."

Gradually, *very* gradually, his depression lifted. Today, he's healthy and happy. He has a real-estate licence, and does consulting work for the Ontario government. He runs five miles a day, rides his bike, walks, and meditates. He's into amateur dramatics. "In the last couple of years with this new health regime," he enthuses, "I've got my self-confidence back, and I'm enjoying it [theatre] so much I may consider turning professional. . . . Now I can acknowledge that I'm quite talented, because I have confidence in myself. I usually play the lead!"

A recent study by the Fraser Institute found that half of Canadians use alternative (also called complementary) therapies, spending almost $4 billion a year in the process. Topping the list were chiropractic work, relaxation techniques, massage, prayer, and herbal therapies. The most common ailments being treated were back and neck problems, headaches, allergies, and arthritis/rheumatism.

Today, many mental health consumers are also trying these alternatives. Weary of conventional Western medicine, which separates body and mind, and treats illnesses in isolation, they're turning to holistic systems, which focus on maintaining overall health and have been practised for centuries.

"In medicine, psychology, psychoanalysis, all these fields, quite often the theories are about illnesses, and not very much about health," says Dr. Jacques Bradwejn, chairman of psychiatry at the University of Ottawa. "Complementary medicines, because they're very comprehensive, health-based approaches, bring that richness and complement really scientific, medical approaches that are disease-based."

Many consumers find alternative approaches more natural than psychiatry. Others may be looking for a spiritual or philosophical approach more in sync with their own belief systems (and there is much to be said for the power of belief in the healing process). And most people appreciate the amount of time and interest practitioners offer, often in sharp contrast to the doctor's office.

Perhaps the most common and powerful factor, however, is choice. The power to be a truly active partner in the healing process.

Despite their growing popularity, alternative medicines are still regarded with caution by the medical profession. A few treatments are slowly finding their way into hospitals and doctors' offices – acupuncture is a good example – but for the most part, physicians aren't well informed about what's out there, and are unlikely to recommend alternative treatments. They usually claim there isn't enough hard science behind it.

Dr. Bradwejn wants to change that. He's made it his mission to put alternative medicines to the scientific test, and to encourage collaboration between practitioners, physicians, and other mental health professionals. In some ways, he's the perfect go-between: a world-renowned researcher, rooted in the scientific method, but keenly interested in what alternative medicines have to offer.

That interest began several years ago. While working at McGill University he made a major discovery: he identified a protein in the brain that can induce panic attacks. Later, while working at the University of Toronto, he learned that a herbal compound used for centuries in the East acted on the same protein system. Dr. Bradwejn was intrigued.

"Here is a system that was discovered ten years ago, which seems to play a role in the cause of panic attacks," he told a CMHA journal, "and here are herbs which have been used for hundreds, even thousands, of years, to treat anxiety and tension, which act on the same system."

By chance, his Toronto office was right next to Chinatown. He ran across the street, spoke with some traditional practitioners, and began organizing a symposium that would introduce doctors and psychiatrists to traditional Chinese medicine, homeopathy, meditation, shamanism, and Ayurvedic medicine. He's been researching alternative treatments ever since.

Dr. Bradwejn will be our informal guide as we describe several of these methods. Although we've divided them into separate categories, some practitioners will recommend *combinations* of treatments that suit your own specific symptoms, circumstances, and personality. Practitioners of traditional Chinese medicine, Ayurvedic medicine, and naturopathy, for example, look at the whole person, and try to find the mix of approaches that will help you most.

A couple of notes before we start.

Alternative and conventional treatments needn't be mutually exclusive. Many people try both. As Britain's Mental Health Foundation concluded after surveying consumers, "Supporting the use of alternative and complementary therapies in mental health is often seen as encouraging people to give up their medication in favour of aromatherapy or massage. The reality for people living and coping with mental health problems is that a range of different things might be helpful at different times – and this includes medication."

However, if you're considering trying alternative treatment, either in conjunction with or instead of meds, see your doctor first. You will need to be monitored.

As with conventional medical treatments, the authors cannot recommend or endorse any alternative treatment for any disorder. Again, only you, in consultation with your doctor, can decide what might work for you.

HERBS

We have been using nature's garden for medicinal purposes for thousands of years. And that tradition has carried over to modern medicines. Many – by Dr. Bradwejn's estimate 40% – of today's drugs have their origin in herbs. The chemical basis of Aspirin, for example, was originally found in white willow bark, and the heart medication digitalis comes from foxglove.

Consumers troubled by the side effects and chemical makeup of psychiatric medications see herbal remedies as more natural, and safe. But that isn't necessarily so. "There are many natural poisons out there," Dr. Bradwejn notes, "and many herbal compounds are not necessarily harmless." In fact, some herbs are extremely potent, with active ingredients that work on the brain in the same way pharmaceuticals do.

Natural products also aren't regulated as rigorously as prescription drugs, and consumers don't always get what the labels claim. The *Toronto Star* newspaper, in an investigation of herbal products, sent ten brands each of garlic, ginseng, and feverfew to a laboratory for analysis. The results were startling: "Some products showed no trace of the active ingredient they promised," the paper reported. "Others delivered far less than the amount printed on their label. Some making no claims registered higher levels than brands with big promises."

The *Star* also noted that in the previous two years, Health Canada had issued warnings about more than a dozen herbal medicines found to contain mercury, arsenic, and other toxins.

Although Health Canada has opened an Office of Natural Health Products, and promises new quality standards and labelling rules, as of publication date there were no Canadian regulations obliging manufacturers to guarantee the purity of their product.

For these reasons, all herbal products should be used with care, and preferably in consultation with an experienced practitioner. Herbalists, naturopaths, practitioners of traditional Chinese or Ayurvedic medicine, and aboriginal healers all use herbs in their treatment plans. Often, they'll prescribe combinations of herbs, tailored to your own symptoms, personality, and overall health. There are dozens of herbal products on the market, and conflicting reports about what each may help treat. A trained practitioner can help make sense of all this.

There is mounting scientific evidence that some herbs *do* have beneficial effects. We'll talk about the most promising ones. But there are many others that fall into the category of "needing more study." That doesn't mean the herbs are worthless, only that the benefits consumers often describe have not been scientifically proven. These include German chamomile, hops, lemon balm, passion flower, and skullcap, all used mainly for anxiety and insomnia. You and your practitioner may decide any one of them is worth trying.

St. John's Wort

This shrubby yellow plant is the best-known and most popular herbal antidepressant. It's also the best researched – enough so that Dr. Bradwejn feels comfortable recommending it to some of his patients. "There's fairly good evidence that St. John's wort can work for *mild to moderate* depression," he says (italics added).

Much of that evidence comes from Europe, where the herb has been widely used for years. In Germany, St. John's wort is the top-selling antidepressant (although it requires a doctor's prescription there). Many published studies have found it works as well as chemical antidepressants, with fewer side effects. It's also cheaper.

No one knows how this herb works, but an active compound called hypericin seems to be involved. Dr. Bradwejn suggests that the most effective products contain a hypericin content of .3% and should be taken in pill form at 300 mg, three times a day. Look for a label that says "standardized preparation," which means the dosage is guaranteed and the contents are free of impurities.

Side effects may include increased sensitivity to sunlight, nausea, dizziness, fatigue, confusion, and dry mouth, but these are usually mild. Sexual dysfunction – a side effect of many synthesized antidepressants – is extremely rare. As with other antidepressants, there may be adverse reactions when taken with other drugs, or during pregnancy. For this reason, you should always let your physician know if you're taking this or any other herbal product.

St. John's wort can take up to two months to work, and its long-term efficacy is not known. It's also not known if St. John's wort works on severe depression. Research will try to answer these questions. Dr. Bradwejn is a scientific adviser on a long-term study of more than three hundred patients conducted by the National Institute of Mental Health in the United States. The study has tracked the progress of severely depressed patients taking either St. John's wort, a placebo, or a standard antidepressant medication. Results are not yet available.

"It's a good precedent," Dr. Bradwejn says of the study, "because if it shows efficacy, it will open the door to do the same thing with many herbal compounds."

The NIMH has also issued an alert warning of "adverse interactions" between St. John's wort and two drugs: one used to treat HIV, and the other used with organ transplants. Consult your doctor before combining any medications with herbal products.

Kava

South Pacific islanders have been using this stuff for a long time – by some accounts, for up to three thousand years. But now it's as close as your local health-food store or pharmacy. Made from the root of the kava tree, it's generally used as a mild sedative for anxiety, and seems not to cause grogginess or to contain the addictive properties associated with prescription benzodiazepines. If you suffer from mild to moderate anxiety, you might consider it as an alternative to an anxiolytic. The standard dose is 100 to 200 mg a day.

A handful of European studies have found it more effective than a placebo. In a recent issue of the *Archives of General Psychiatry*, a Canadian review of research on herbal remedies found that "several human clinical trials suggest that kava products standardized for kavalactone content (70%) may be beneficial in the management of anxiety and tension of nonpsychotic origin."

Dr. Bradwejn has started his own study of kava, but until the results are in, he will say only that it may be effective for mild generalized anxiety. "It's been shown to have anxiety-reducing properties, but very broadly. We don't know whether it's anxiety to a significant level that would constitute an anxiety disorder."

The risks associated with long-term use, or of combining kava with prescription drugs, are also unknown; the *Archives* article notes that long-term use at high doses may cause scaling of the skin. Kava may also increase the effects of alcohol, so it's best to avoid alcoholic drinks while taking this product.

Valerian Root

This herb has long been used throughout the world for its sedative properties. People who have trouble sleeping often find a pill or two works well at bedtime.

Research on valerian, however, is limited. The *Archives of General Psychiatry* article referred to above found that "human clinical studies of valerian confirm a mild sedative effect," but cautioned "there is no evidence to suggest that valerian is superior to existing hypnotic medications or other treatments for insomnia." Mind you, the article cited no evidence suggesting it is *inferior.*

The standard dosage is 150 to 300 mg of valerian extract (0.8% valeric acid), taken at bedtime. Again, it may be a safer alternative to tranquillizers, with fewer side effects. One warning though: valerian really stinks. Hold your nose when you open the bottle, and prepare for an overpowering blue cheese smell to fill the room.

Ginkgo

This ancient deciduous tree produces a hip new herb, made popular by claims that it sharpens the mind. Indeed, millions of people take it every year. Controlled studies suggest it can help with memory loss caused by Alzheimers and other dementias. Although there's less evidence that ginkgo helps healthy people, many who take it swear this herb improves their memory, concentration, energy levels, and mood.

The usual dose is 40 mg, taken three times daily. Side effects are uncommon, but may include headache, gastrointestinal upset, or restlessness. There have also been very rare reports that ginkgo can thin the blood or impair clotting, so caution is advised for people currently taking anticoagulants.

OTHER COMPOUNDS

Right next to the herbs on the store shelf, you'll find a couple of other natural products that research suggests can give your mental health a boost. One comes from fish oil; the other from your own body.

SAM-e

Move over, Prozac; SAM-e (pronounced *sammy*) is the latest darling of the mental health market, making the headlines in *Newsweek*, *Time*, *USA Today*, and elsewhere. It's also one of the hottest-selling dietary supplements on the North American market.

Like St. John's wort, SAM-e (or S-Adenosylmethionine) became popular first in Europe, where it's widely used as an alternative to synthetic antidepressants. But SAM-e isn't a herb; it's a compound produced in the body, thought to work naturally on the very same neurotransmitters that Prozac and other drugs target synthetically.

Dozens of small European clinical trials have found SAM-e works well, even for major depression. It also works quickly, and with few side effects. Still, many North American researchers – including Dr. Bradwejn – are reluctant to endorse it until larger, more rigorous studies have been conducted.

SAM-e's biggest drawback is its price. It costs $1 to $2 per pill – and the usual dosage is eight pills a day. It doesn't take much math to figure out that many consumers will find the cost prohibitive. In fact, SAM-e is more expensive than many prescription drugs.

The usual dose is 1600–2000 mg, taken in pill form. Side effects, although rare and mild, may include stomach upset, headaches, or drowsiness. It should also be avoided by people with bipolar affective disorder, because SAM-e could trigger a manic episode.

Omega-3 Fatty Acids

You've probably given very little thought to the influence of fish oil in your life. But many researchers now believe the omega-3 fatty acids contained in fish such as salmon, mackerel, sardines, and tuna play an important role in our moods and behaviour; low levels may even contribute to the development of disorders like depression, bipolar disorder, anxiety, and schizophrenia.

Though just two servings of fish per week probably provides enough of these fatty acids, our North American diets tend to be low in them. And population studies show that as consumption of omega-3 falls, depression rates rise. Researchers are now looking for scientific evidence that fish-oil supplements – available in capsules in most health-food stores – can ease symptoms of many mental disorders.

So far, the early evidence has yet to be replicated. But one recent U.S. pilot study has attracted a lot of attention. This double-blind controlled study monitored thirty out-patients with bipolar disorder; they'd all had at least one manic or hypomanic episode in the past year. Fourteen were given fish-oil capsules; the other sixteen received placebo capsules of olive oil. During the four-month study, the group taking fish oil had a significantly longer period of remission of symptoms.

"Omega 3 Fatty acids used as an adjunctive treatment in bipolar disorder resulted in significant symptom reduction and a better outcome when compared with placebo," the authors reported. "The striking difference in relapse rates and response appeared to be highly clinically significant."

The only side effect was mild gastrointestinal upset, and most subjects were happy to take the capsules. Note, though, that the fish oil was used as an *adjunct* treatment; most patients in the study were also on mood stabilizers. There's still no solid evidence that the fish oil works on its own.

"The only way I would use omega-3s by themselves is in someone with an extremely mild form of the illness where treatment is almost optional," lead author Dr. Andrew Stoll later told the *Psychiatric Times*. "Otherwise, we use omega-3s as an adjunct."

Dr. Stoll is now conducting a larger study of omega-3 and bipolar disorder. Other clinical trials are looking at the effect these fatty acids have on depression and schizophrenia. Dr. Bradwejn, meanwhile, says the published research on fish oil is promising. "It seems to have some effect," he says. "It's been established in very high-standard publications."

VITAMINS/NUTRITION

We are what we eat – and that applies to the mind as well as the body. There's considerable research linking nutrition with mood, and linking specific psychiatric disorders with vitamin deficiencies.

Folic acid, for example, is a B vitamin often found to be low in people hospitalized for depression and schizophrenia. "In medical patients psychiatric symptoms occur more frequently, and in psychiatric patients symptoms are more severe in those with folate deficiency than in those with normal levels," one Canadian study notes. Foods rich in folic acid include green leafy vegetables, citrus fruits, whole grains, beans, and legumes, as well as poultry, pork, and liver. Supplementary doses are sometimes used as cheap, safe adjunct treatments, particularly for depression. You can buy folic acid in pill form at most pharmacies and health-food stores.

Other research has focused on an essential amino acid called tryptophan; low levels of this have been shown to lower serotonin levels, which have been linked with lower moods. Even in healthy people, studies have shown that when tryptophan levels are rapidly depleted, mood tends to drop. When this is done for research purposes to people in remission from depression, rates of relapse go up. Tryptophan supplements are often used to treat seasonal affective disorder. They're also prescribed occasionally as an adjunct treatment for depression or anxiety, although doctors don't all agree that it works. Tryptophan is not available over the counter; you'll need a doctor's prescription. You can also boost levels by eating protein-rich foods like meat, fish, eggs, dairy products, soy, and lentils.

On a more general level, many consumers report that sticking to a healthy diet of regular meals is helpful. This is especially tough to do if you're depressed; lifting a spoon, let alone cooking a meal, can feel like way too much work. We recall the advice of one young man at a meeting of the Mood Disorders Association. He'd just recovered from a severe depression. "You've got to force yourself to eat," he said. "Get out of bed, fill that bowl with cereal, and make yourself eat."

Nutritionists, dietitians, and naturopaths can help you improve your diet and recommend vitamin and mineral supplements. Some even specialize in mental health. They may also look at your sugar and caffeine consumption, and the mix of protein and carbohydrates in your diet. If you want more information, there are plenty of books on the nutritional approach to mental health; check your bookstore, library, or local self-help group.

Orthomolecular Therapy

Proponents of this therapy take the view that even serious disorders like schizophrenia are caused (or aggravated) by vitamin deficiencies and nutritional imbalances. Therapy involves prescribing megadoses of vitamins, minerals, and/or amino acids to restore balance. The prescribed diet reduces processed foods, adds natural foods, and is modified after testing for food allergies.

There's lots of anecdotal evidence that this works; one of its high-profile supporters is Canadian actress Margot Kidder, who has been diagnosed with bipolar disorder. She credits orthomolecular therapy with helping her maintain her mental health.

Canada is also home to one of the field's founders and leading researchers, Dr. Abram Hoffer. Now in his eighties, he's been treating people with schizophrenia for several decades.

The medical community does not endorse this approach, and notes that high doses of some vitamins can be harmful. Dr. Bradwejn, however, believes orthomolecular therapy warrants more study. "It's certainly of interest," he says. "But double-blind randomized control trials are missing. They're necessary. That doesn't mean it won't work for some people. But more and more consumers want to know: is there proof."

EXERCISE

Whether it's a walk, jog, swim, or game of tennis, there's little doubt that exercise is good for both body *and* soul. Exercise releases those natural mood elevators called endorphins (the stuff that produces a "runner's high") and lowers levels of cortisol, a hormone linked with stress. It can also help psychologically, by increasing your sense of self-worth and providing a welcome diversion from unpleasant thoughts and feelings.

Research has repeatedly shown that exercise helps people overcome depression, either on its own or with other treatments. "No controlled study has ever found exercise to be an ineffective primary or adjunctive treatment for mild to moderate depression," according to one recent review of studies on exercise and mental health written by researchers at the University of Manitoba and published in the journal *Professional Psychology*. The paper notes that both aerobic workouts (walking, running) and non-aerobic ones (weight-training) are effective; they're also relatively cheap and accessible, with long-lasting benefits.

Regular physical activity may also help people with anxiety disorders. Some research suggests it can reduce psychotic symptoms and hallucinations, and improve social functioning, for people with schizophrenia. In both these areas, the paper concluded more research is needed to confirm these effects.

You don't have to run a marathon to enjoy some of the benefits. Tai Qi is a series of gentle, meditative exercises practised for centuries in China; an Australian study found that people who had completed a two-month course later reported less stress, anxiety, and depression.

Even something as simple as a daily walk or yoga session can be therapeutic. People report that these activities help ease the stiffness associated with some antipsychotic medications. They also get you out of the house, let you take some control over the disorder. Try some activity you once enjoyed – even if it seems impossible to enjoy *anything* now. And remember – it's always a good idea to check with your doctor before you start a new exercise program.

ACUPUNCTURE

This technique has been practised in China for more than two thousand years. Acupuncturists gently insert thin needles at precise points on the skin to alleviate specific conditions. It's based on the belief that *Qi* – or energy – courses through the body along certain pathways, or meridians. When this vital energy becomes imbalanced, or the pathways become blocked, illness results. Acupuncture improves health by removing the blockages and restoring balance.

Acupuncture is gaining acceptance in Western medicine; many hospitals now use it to treat headaches, back pain, and substance abuse. Recent research suggests it can help treat depression as well.

A pilot study at the University of Arizona used acupuncture to treat thirty-three middle-aged women with mild to moderate depression. After eight weeks of treatment by a trained practitioner, about two-thirds of the women experienced full remission of symptoms. (To rule out the placebo effect, one group of women was first given acupuncture to treat *other* symptoms – such as back pain – without their knowledge. These women had lower rates of remission. They were later given the depression-specific treatment.)

"Results from this small sample suggest that acupuncture can provide significant symptom relief in depression, at rates comparable to those of psychotherapy or pharmacotherapy," wrote John Allen, lead author of the paper in which the study's findings were published.

The acupuncture was also well tolerated by the women, with no side effects, and with lower dropout rates than medication or psychotherapy generally produce. A one-year follow-up is now underway; at the half-way point, the relapse rate was comparable to other treatments.

Dr. Allen is also conducting a larger study to try to replicate the pilot study results. If you want to consider treatment by this method, he suggests you find an experienced, certified acupuncturist with training in traditional Chinese medicine. You'll also want to ensure that only disposable needles are used. You may experience tingling or numbness while the needle is in place, but many people find the experience relaxing, even falling asleep on the table.

MEDITATION/RELAXATION

Just *relax*. . . . In our stressed-out modern world, that advice is easier to give than it is to follow. Thankfully, there are now several techniques designed to help us relax – and they seem to work with a number of disorders, including anxiety and depression. They may not *cure* us, but they can certainly help us cope better.

One very simple technique is called progressive relaxation therapy, or PRT. Lying on the floor, you focus on different muscle groups, tensing and then relaxing them. Often, you start with the feet, and move up the body, tensing and relaxing, until you reach the face. To finish the session, you tense and relax your entire body. The result is an overall feeling of calm.

Meditation is another form of relaxation, which may be beneficial for some mood and anxiety disorders. "It seems there's evidence it could help," Dr. Bradwejn says.

There are several techniques – walking, sitting, lying down, using mantras, chants, or candles – but the one that's gaining popularity as a treatment for depression or anxiety is called Mindfulness Meditation. Though it involves learning relaxation techniques, it could aptly be described as an approach to everyday living that helps people manage stress by becoming aware of their thoughts and feelings.

Developed at the University of Massachusetts Medical Center by Dr. Jon Kabat-Zinn, it's been used there to treat (and study) pain and psychiatric disorders. One study followed up on a group of people with panic and anxiety disorders three years after they'd learned the technique. It concluded that "stress reduction intervention based on mindfulness meditation can have long-term beneficial effects in the treatment of people diagnosed with anxiety disorders."

Here in Canada, psychologist Zindel Segal has begun researching a program that integrates mindfulness meditation with cognitive therapy for use in the treatment of recurrent depression. It's called mindfulness-based cognitive therapy (MBCT). People are taught to become more aware of their thoughts and feelings, and to relate to those thoughts and feelings in nonjudgmental ways. These skills can be applied for a lifetime; early research shows they can help reduce the risk of relapse.

"The mindfulness training becomes something that is done on an everyday basis, and that's where you get the protection," Dr. Segal says. "Because that lets you see small mood changes, and lets you do something about them before they grow into large problems."

In one study by Dr. Segal and others (soon to be published), researchers monitored 145 patients with recurrent depression who'd recently recovered from a major episode. Some continued with just their usual treatment, while others were also trained in MBCT. Over the course of a year, the recurrence rates were significantly lower for the group receiving MBCT.

If you're interested in meditation or relaxation techniques, there are lots of books and tapes available – Dr. Kabat-Zinn has written several. Some types of meditation are spiritually based; others are simple exercises designed to clear the mind. Basic meditation courses are offered in many communities.

SPIRITUALITY

This is a tough one to test scientifically, based as it is on our own individual belief systems. But a few researchers are taking a stab at it, and early evidence suggests that religious beliefs *can* make a difference to both our physical and mental health. What seems to matter most is not religious *practice* (church attendance or prayer) but something called *intrinsic religiosity* – the spiritual beliefs we build into our daily lives.

"A certain type of religiosity seems to help speed up recovery or the extent of recovery," Dr. Bradwejn notes. "People who have an innate spirituality, which could even be in very broad terms, not scriptural or theological – especially if they believe in some supreme system or God as a loving entity – do better."

He cites one rigorous scientific trial led by Dr. Harold Koenig at Duke University Medical Center, and published in the *American Journal of Psychiatry*. It looked at how religious belief affected remission of depression in 111 older, hospitalized patients. After their discharge, the patients were given four psychiatric interviews over forty-seven weeks. In that time, 54% of them achieved remission. After controlling for other variables (physical health, treatment, demographic and psychosocial factors), they found religiosity did make a significant difference. "Depressed patients with higher intrinsic religiosity scores had more rapid remissions than patients with lower scores. . . . In this study, greater intrinsic religiosity independently predicted shorter time to remission."

BIOFEEDBACK

Biofeedback is something like a language – one that allows you to communicate with your body. Sensors attached to the skin monitor things like muscle tension, pulse, and body temperature. Physical changes are translated into an audible tone, or a visual signal on a monitor. People then learn to control the signal or sound by relaxing, breathing, altering thoughts – whatever it takes.

Research has shown that biofeedback does work; people can train themselves to ease tension, reduce headaches and neck pain. One U.S. study tested its effectiveness on 150 children with anxiety difficulties. Half the group learned biofeedback techniques to reduce symptoms of anxiety, while the other group received no intervention. After six weeks, the biofeedback group reported – and exhibited – far fewer symptoms than the control group.

Biofeedback is rapidly gaining acceptance in the medical community; the Canadian Psychiatric Association now recognizes its use as an adjunct treatment for anxiety states and insomnia.

OTHERS

Of course, we've barely skimmed the surface here. There are scores more treatments, not yet well studied, but worthy of scientific research. Many consumers swear by these other alternative practices and therapies. So we encourage you to do your own research; read and talk to fellow consumers about what's worked for them. Here's just a brief look at what's out there.

Aromatherapy: Anyone who's sniffed a bouquet of flowers, or breathed in the aroma of freshly baked cookies, knows that scent can make us feel good. Aromatherapy works on the principle that scent elicits responses in the brain, and therefore affects emotions. Lavender, for example, is supposed to be calming; rosemary, stimulating. Essential oils can be used in massage, in the bath, or through an air freshener or diffuser. A qualified aromatherapist will blend oils for therapeutic effect.

Art/dance/music: These creative outlets can be used as therapy, to reduce depression, anxiety, or stress, and to help people explore their emotions. Some research suggests that music can even work physiologically, affecting blood pressure and heart rates. Doctors may refer patients to qualified art, dance, or music therapists.

Homeopathy: This approach involves the use of minute quantities of highly diluted substances, about two thousand of which are now available. There's much debate about how – and if – these tiny doses work, and the medical community remains highly sceptical. Nonetheless, homeopathy has been popular in India and Europe for decades – and has been used to treat a number of mental health problems, including depression, anxiety, and bipolar disorder. Homeopathic remedies are closely tailored to each individual patient (which makes them hard to study scientifically); doctors are highly trained and holistic in approach, and will do a thorough consultation before prescribing treatment.

Massage therapy: Massage loosens tight muscles and joints, but it may also relax your mind. It's been practised for centuries as a way of improving not only physical but also mental and emotional health. (If you've ever placed yourself in skilled hands, you'll know how effective a tension-reliever massage can be.) Several techniques are now popular: Swedish, deep tissue, acupressure, Shiatsu, to name just a few. So it's worth asking around or trying more than one.

Therapeutic touch: Practitioners send healing energy into the recipient by moving their hands on or near the skin. This has been found to reduce anxiety in hospitalized patients, including psychiatric patients. It's a gentle, quiet, calming technique, often practised by nurses; look for a trained practitioner.

SOME PARTING ADVICE

If you're interested in alternative treatments, it may be worthwhile to find a medical doctor who will support, and even share, your interest. Dr. Bradwejn, for example, has found that his research into alternative practices has changed his own clinical approach. He looks at mental disorder in a multi-dimensional way, considering all the possible contributing factors. His focus is on achieving health (including emotional and spiritual health) and figuring out the barriers that may be getting in the way. "The goal is health," he says. "What's health? We – the patient and I – define it in more precise terms, and look at the illness as a barrier to that. . . . The context is different; it's removing the barriers to health, having discussed what health is and what the goals will be."

Dr. Bradwejn offers the following advice to anyone considering alternative treatment for a mental disorder:

1. Consult your doctor. It's important to know what the problem is before you start any treatment. Rather than trying to self-diagnose, see your GP or psychiatrist first, then decide what treatments – alternative *and/or* conventional – might work best.
2. Do some research. Find out what's been shown to work, or not work. We've provided a very brief overview here, but there's lots more information out there. Weigh the risks and potential benefits of each alternative treatment, and the risks of rejecting conventional treatments.
3. See a specialist. "I would advise not to self-treat," Dr. Bradwejn says. "Not to run to the store and take a herbal compound or a vitamin. If you want to go that route . . . go the whole way. See an acupuncturist or a Chinese doctor or Ayurvedic doctor. Then you get the whole package. You get the evaluation according to that system. You get some advice."

   Look for a qualified practitioner who will provide references and describe to you his or her training and experience. This is especially important, because many alternative practices are unregulated; anyone can claim to be an expert. Ask around, check with the associations that many alternative practitioners have formed. Ethical practitioners know their limits and won't promise miracle cures.

4. Set goals. Just as with conventional medicines, it's important to gauge, and expect, improvement. If this isn't happening, try another alternative and/or conventional treatment. "For example," Dr. Bradwejn says, "I have depression. I'll set a goal of being well in two months. If that's not coming about, then okay, I'll turn the page and go for the antidepressant. . . . Quite often, what I see is people who keep trying this and trying that. They never set a goal or re-evaluate."

5. Consider costs. Unfortunately, you'll have to pay for most alternative treatments from your own pocket. And they don't work overnight. So discuss with the practitioner how many treatments may be required, over what length of time, and then do the math. Make sure you can afford to see the treatment through. Also, if you're spending vast quantities of money without noticeable improvement, look elsewhere. Check with your private and provincial healthcare plans; some treatments, such as massage, may be covered with a doctor's note.

The path to wellness is rarely as straightforward as popping a vitamin or drinking some herbal tea. So if you're looking for a quick fix, you probably won't find it here. The people who benefit most are the ones who incorporate these practices into a new and healthier approach to life. As William Boyd's story illustrated at the beginning of this chapter, changing the way you care for *yourself* can change your life. This is the very essence, and beauty, of alternative medicines: they help us to help ourselves. They show us that our bodies and minds not only respond to care, but deserve it too.

STEVE'S STORY

I was born December 16, 1964, in Sault Ste. Marie, Ontario, to the late Veronica Jocko. She was of Status Indian descent from the Algonquins of Golden Lake First Nation, which I am also a band member of. I am not too sure who my father is, but have recently found a biological sister who lives in Vanier, Ontario.

It all started with my biological mother. When she was young, she was forced to attend a residential school in the town of Spanish, where sexual abuse was a reality and the school's mission was to wipe out aboriginal culture. As a result, my mother developed alcoholism and mental health problems. Subsequently, when I was a baby, the Children's Aid Society took me and my sister away and adopted us to separate families. I was raised in a white home, and I knew nothing of my aboriginal past. I was never fully adopted. The Children's Aid Society's mandate is to protect, but I grew up in a very dysfunctional alcoholic and drug-addicted home which has affected my entire life. I am currently trying to heal from this and lead a normal life.

By the age of thirteen, I was getting into drugs and alcohol. I felt out of place and different. Growing up was very hard, because for me racism was an everyday occurrence.

In 1975, my adoptive father introduced me to the sport of amateur boxing, which would later consume my life for more than twenty years. Originally I took the sport for self-defence, but I never had to use it. By the time I had finished my amateur career, I had accumulated more than 150 amateur bouts, along with eight national titles and attendance at more than twenty international tournaments. Most notable were the 1986 World Championships, where I placed in the top eight, and the 1986 Commonwealth Games, where I earned a bronze medal.

In 1984 I tried college, enrolling in Sault College's mechanical engineering program. While I was there, I was training for the 1988 Canadian Olympic team that would compete in Seoul, South Korea. Boxing was my first priority and it took up all of my time. I couldn't juggle school and sports, so I had to make a choice. I decided to drop out of school in 1987, a year before my graduation.

I trained hard every day, aiming for the Olympics, but my heavy drinking hurt my chances. In 1987 I lost my spot on the National "A" Team. In 1988 I lost in both the national championships and the Olympic trials and left the sport bitter, depressed, and totally disappointed in myself. This was probably one of the lowest points of my life, and this is when my drinking problem grew into full-blown alcoholism. Shortly afterward, I was on the brink of kidney failure because of a suicide attempt, and I knew I needed to seek help. It was not because I wanted to die, it was that all I wanted to do was to get rid of all that pain that I had inside of me. Suicide, I thought, was the only option.

Western methods had failed me, so I went to see a native addiction counsellor. I was referred to a native drug-and-alcohol treatment centre (Weendaahmaagin) in Thunder Bay, and that's where I was eventually able to arrest my alcoholism. Weendaahmaagin's holistic approach to healing (viewing the physical, mental, spiritual, and emotional elements as connected to each other and ideally in balance) provided me with links to my past; links that began to answer my identity questions and give me a sense of meaning. Finally I began to learn who Steve Beaupré was all about, and especially about being an Indian.

After completing my treatment at Weendaahmaagin, I was thirsty for more knowledge about my aboriginal roots. I was able to satisfy that thirst at Sault College in 1991 by enrolling in the Native Community Worker/Addiction Counsellor program, and since then my life has never been the same.

I competed again in amateur boxing, but this time I was clean and sober. I had never set my goals at making the 1992 Olympic team; it was the farthest thing from my mind. I won the 1991 National Championships and Pan American trials, but would not compete in the 1991 Pan Am Games because of politics. The politics in the sport took away that drive or spark I needed to secure a spot on the 1992 Olympic team. By this time school was my primary focus and boxing was secondary. I lost at both the 1992 Nationals and 1992 Olympic Box Offs and was able to walk away from the sport by putting to sleep the demons that had haunted me since 1988. I could now accept that it was not meant to be and move on with my life.

I experienced a lot of personal growth while I was a student at Sault College. The program's Native component taught me so much about my people and the culture. I have been working in the Native community since 1993, which has been one long learning experience for me. Healing is about learning and understanding. Most of my life I hated Native people, but I learned that was because I had always hated myself for being an Indian. Today I can look in the mirror and say that I love that person looking back at me.

I'm currently working at the Enaahtig Healing Lodge and Learning Centre in Victoria Harbour, Ontario, where I fill the position of Program Coordinator. I supervise a staff of six, and my primary responsibility is the delivery of programs and services offered at the lodge. I also teach in the Native Community and Social Development course at Georgian College.

Sometimes I have to pinch myself, because it seems like a wonderful dream. When I turned to a native approach to healing, my life totally changed. I went back to college and earned a diploma; I've enjoyed steady job satisfaction; I'm happily married to my true love, Tracy, and we have three beautiful children, Cody, Stephanie, and Hunter. I'm proud to say that I've been clean and sober for eleven years. I am currently learning about the Anishnabi culture from probably one of the last true oral teachers. In order to follow the native culture, one must be totally clean from all drugs and alcohol. I am blessed today with so much; I have been given a second chance. I will end by saying this: "I may not be what I want to be. And I'm not what I ought to be. But thanks to the Creator I'm not what I used to be!"

Meegwetch *("Thank you")*.

CHAPTER TEN

Suicide

"Suicide is a tragic and perplexing phenomenon that eventually, in one way or another, touches the lives of most Canadians."

— *Task Force on Suicide in Canada, 1994*

Like most people who decide to kill themselves, Jennifer was not convinced she truly wanted to die. She knew only that living had become too hard, that she no longer had the strength to carry its burden. Suicide, she finally concluded, "was the only way I could see of stopping it or changing it."

She was just sixteen years old at the time.

"There are so many things that went into it," she recalls. "Certainly I had a lot of self-hatred. And I think what really kept me from being able to get *out* of being suicidal is that I had no ability . . . to talk to anyone about my feelings."

In retrospect, there were signs this young woman was at risk. Her marks at school had taken a sharp drop, she was abusing drugs, there were constant troubles at home – troubles never openly discussed. Her family didn't like to show their feelings or express emotions. So she didn't.

"Everything was inside and had no way of getting out. I started feeling increasingly desperate.

"The final straw was losing connection with my boyfriend at the time. It was actually on Valentine's Day. I often refer to it as my own little St. Valentine's Day Massacre."

And so she did it. Took a handful of prescription pills and shoved them into her mouth. She was rushed to hospital where an emergency team induced vomiting to clear her system. Almost everyone close to her reacted in horror to what she had done – except for one friend.

"The thing that was most important to me at the time, the person who responded best of anyone, was the friend who said, 'I'm glad you're alive. And if you're feeling that way again, call me'," she remembers. "It was just so simple."

Had she known of that support *prior* to her attempt, Jennifer thinks she might not have swallowed the pills at all. It was, she says, what she needed most.

"Having someone I could talk to and share feelings with, someone who just valued me."

Over time, Jennifer dealt with the many issues that had pushed her toward suicide. The things that seemed so insurmountable back then were eventually resolved. Now forty-one, with joyous eyes and a generous smile, she appears to revel in life – a feeling enhanced by the knowledge that she's lucky to be here.

"It was pretty pivotal for me when I realized, much later in my life, that I was having a moment when I was just totally delighted to be alive. And that really has affected the way that I perceive suicide."

Suicide is *the* last taboo. It is a topic rarely openly discussed. We regard it as bleak, desolate, unspeakable. A sacrilege.

Which is astonishing, given the statistics.

In 1997, the official number of suicides in this country was 3,681. That's ten Canadians, young and old, rich and poor, ending their lives every single day of the year. Many more harm themselves with suicidal intent. In fact, it's estimated that for every suicide, at least one hundred other attempts will take place.

Yet, for the most part, we cling to silence. It's something that only happens to *other* people.

We should reassess that view. An Alberta organization that offers suicide prevention workshops – LivingWorks Education Inc. – has surveyed more than fifty thousand Canadians. It found, in virtually every part of the country, that 66% of us know of a friend, family member, or acquaintance who has taken their own life. Clearly, suicide is not as distant as we might like to believe. And the numbers from Statistics Canada confirm it. In 1997 there were 3,026 deaths from traffic accidents in Canada, 440 deaths from homicide, and *3,681* from suicide.

The total number of suicides is greater than deaths due to traffic accidents and homicides *combined*. It is one of the top ten causes of death in this country.

A COMPLEX ACT

Rule Number One: Suicide is complex. It is only rarely prompted by a single event we can look to as the "cause."

"You sometimes get caught up looking for that one thing that's responsible," says Toronto suicidologist Ian Dawe, "and in fact there are multiple causes to each and every suicide."

"Be very careful not to assume that suicidal acts are a consequence of crisis," warns Dr. Bryan Tanney. "Suicide doesn't just happen because of something that happened yesterday." A professor of psychiatry at the University of Calgary with a quarter-century's experience in the field, Tanney (and other clinicians) says the path toward suicide usually follows one of these two routes.

- The person who ends their life has endured countless painful stressors over a long period of time. Then, a final straw – and it can be a small one – pushes them into what is sometimes called "the suicide zone."

- The individual has previously been able to draw on their coping skills and deal with life's many obstacles. This time, they are unable to muster, perhaps even locate, those skills. Their "resiliency" fails them.

Neither situation presents us with a tidy relationship between cause and effect. "Another way [of looking at suicide] is the *Titanic* analogy," explains Dr. Tanney. "Did it sink because of the iceberg or the faulty rivets? Or maybe because the *California* just did not listen."

A century ago, French sociologist Émile Durkheim attempted to answer the same perplexing question. Why do people end their lives? His landmark work, *Le Suicide*, put the act under a psychosocial microscope in an exhaustive search for clues. His work examined race, religion, class, marital status, mental disorder, sex, age, alcohol consumption – virtually every psychological, geographical, or socio-economic category you could imagine. No possible relationship was considered too remote to explore – including the latitude and weather.

It was an exhaustive work. And a productive one. For *Le Suicide* demonstrated, a century ago, something the vast body of work since then has confirmed: suicide is complex.

The most varied and even the most contradictory events of life may equally serve as pretexts for suicide. This suggests that none of them is the specific cause. Could we perhaps at least ascribe causality to those qualities known to be common to all?

Had Durkheim been familiar with the modern language of suicidology – the scientific field he pioneered – he would likely have used different words: "Suicide is multifactorial. But could we at least nail down some risk factors?"

RISK FACTORS/PROTECTIVE FACTORS

Studies of people who end their lives, and of people who attempt suicide or think about it frequently, show us that there are risk factors. These are characteristics found in a significant number of people who contemplate, attempt, or complete suicide. Being male, for example, is a risk factor: more men than women kill themselves (the ratio in Canada is roughly four to one). Being a First Nations male is an even greater risk factor. Having limited social supports is a risk factor. Substance abuse or dependence is a risk factor.

Conversely, there are protective factors that seem to insulate people from suicidal behaviour. Having a strong religious faith is a protective factor. Having good physical health is a protective factor. Having a supportive friend is a protective factor.

Suicide occurs when the burden of risk factors becomes so crushing that the protective factors no longer offer an escape route.

"The act arises," clarifies Dr. Tanney, "because at that moment suicide offers the best solution for them based on the problem and the capacities, resources, or options which they can bring to resolving it. It may be overwhelming risk or it may be inadequate or paralyzed protection."

But it is important to point out that risk (or protective) factors do not *predict* how an individual will behave.

"We know that people who have had traumatic childhood experiences are more likely to commit suicide," explains suicidologist Dr. Alain LeSage of Montreal. "These are risk factors. Yet . . . the majority of people who have had traumatic childhood experiences *don't* kill themselves."

To put risk factors in context, think of teen driving. We know that as a group adolescent males tend to have more car accidents. Therefore we could say that being a teenaged male is a risk factor for car crashes (which is why their insurance rates are often higher). On an *individual* basis, however, we cannot predict with certainty whether any one teenager will get into an accident.

Certain factors, though, are riskier than others. Drinking and driving carries a greater risk than merely being a teenaged boy. Speeding is a risk factor. And when those risk factors coincide – a drunken teenager behind the wheel of a speeding car – the risk of a smash-up increases.

The same thing applies to suicide. And the people most at risk are those who've already attempted the act.

"Prior suicidal behaviour [PSB] is, bar none, the most significantly demonstrated risk factor," says Calgary's Dr. Tanney. "Numerous studies indicate that persons with PSB complete suicide at a rate approximately forty times that of the general population. This data holds in every culture and nation studied."

Yet even this data is not as grim as it may sound. Because more than 90% of those who have made an attempt do *not* go on to suicide. Meaning most of them are open to help.

"The vast majority of those who self-harm do not want to die," says Dr. Tanney. "So they are relieved to find themselves alive, and hopefully in some sort of care environment where safety and problem-solving can occur."

Not surprisingly, certain mental disorders are also risk factors, with depression and schizophrenia high on the list. A 1994 Task Force Report on Suicide in Canada pointed out that "as a group, people who have been diagnosed with clinically severe depression or some other psychiatric disorder face a statistically higher risk of suicide than the general population. However, existing evidence indicates that no single determinant (including psychiatric disorder) is either necessary or sufficient to bring about suicide, but that each suicide involves the complex interaction of various factors."

In other words, avoid the temptation to simplify cause and effect. There are a multitude of reasons *why* someone with a diagnosis of schizophrenia might end their life – and few are directly related to active psychosis.

"Suicide in this population," states the report, "is rarely attributable to florid psychotic symptoms (hallucinations, delusions); it is more likely to occur in periods of remission or improved functioning. Several studies have indicated that depression and hopelessness are important factors in suicides by persons with schizophrenia, supporting the view that suicide in this population tends to be a planned action."

So it can't be assumed that, on its own, medication to treat the disorder will make the risk vanish. Someone with a diagnosis of schizophrenia may end their life because of chronic unemployment, poverty, isolation, stigmatization. The disorder was a factor in the suicide, but not the sole cause.

THE SIGNS

So how do you know? How can you tell if someone may be at serious risk of suicide?

"Someone talking about suicide is the clearest sign that we know of," says Montreal's Dr. Alain LeSage. "That's absolute. It should *always* be taken seriously."

"You've got to always take it seriously when somebody talks about it," echoes suicidologist Dr. Paul Links. "You have to listen to that."

There is tremendous consensus on that point. When someone talks about killing themselves, they are usually serious. And they're talking because they hope that someone will listen to them.

George Chuvalo learned this lesson in the most painful way possible. The former champion heavyweight boxer has lost four family members – three sons and his wife – to suicide. During a 1999 speech in Toronto to raise suicide awareness, he revealed that the warning signs had been there.

"The one common denominator in all of those," he said with regret, "was that they *told* me. And I diminished that. I said, 'It can't happen.' When people talk about committing suicide, you have to listen."

The data on this is clear.

"Somewhere between 50% and 70% of people who harm themselves give clear and explicit messages that they're going to do it," says Dr. Tanney. Messages, he says, which are not subtle. "They say, 'I'm going to kill myself.' Or, 'I'd be better off if I were dead.' Or, 'I'm not going to be here tomorrow.'

Or, 'Life isn't worth living.' And they give the messages more than once, and they give them to more than one person."

Suicidologists believe these statements are an invitation from the person in distress; an invitation for someone within earshot to offer some help. Problem is, many people are so uncomfortable with the topic of suicide that they would rather not address it. That unease, say authorities, must be overcome.

"When you hear them talking about it," says Dr. Tanney, "your first and major obligation is to bite the bullet, grit your teeth, do whatever you need to do, and say, 'I just heard you say that. I want to clarify what I heard. Are you telling me that you are actually thinking of suicide?' Asking that question, that single question, is the most critical thing that we would like to put forward in the community." He pauses, then repeats emphatically: "Have the courage to ask the question." Ask in a non-judgmental and caring way.

That question can be crucial, because almost every suicidal person is torn between two overwhelming, conflicting urges: the desire to live and the desire to die.

Suicidologists describe this as ambivalence – which seems almost too soft a word given the anguish involved. But the person vacillates – often frequently – between the two options. Viewed in this light, their indecision can be seen as an opportunity, a chance to tip the scales.

Unfortunately, not everyone will express their suicidal thoughts, nor can every suicide be prevented. But there is widespread agreement that when an individual displays the following signs, used by LivingWorks Education Inc. in workshops, it's time to show concern:

When the person *talks* of: escape
having no future
being alone, damaged, helpless
suicide or death[*]
planning for suicide[*]

When the person *feels:*	desperate*
	disconnected
	hopeless
When the *situation* involves:	relationship problems
	work problems/failing grades
	trouble with the law*
	family disruption
	sexual or physical abuse
With *physical changes* like:	lack of interest/pleasure in all things*
	lack of physical energy/disturbed sleep*
	loss of sexual interest/loss of appetite
With *behaviours* like:	alcohol/drug abuse
	fighting/lawbreaking
	emotional outbursts
	dropping out
	prior suicidal behaviour
	putting affairs in order*

* indicates imminent risk

These signs do not necessarily mean the person is going to kill themselves. But they do mean it's time to express concern, particularly if the individual displays one or more behaviours marked as "imminent risk."

And the most effective intervention, agree suicidologists, is to get the person talking. Because one of the most effective prevention strategies involves *listening* to the suicidal person, attempting to understand the immense pain they are living with, letting them know they are not alone.

Some people fear that by talking about suicide openly they may somehow plant the idea or encourage the person to follow through with the act. It's fiction. Dr. Paul Links, head of the Arthur Sommer Rotenberg Chair in Suicide Studies at the University of Toronto – the only research chair in suicide in North America – says the opposite is true.

"This is the old myth that not to say anything is the way to protect the person. It's really the other way around. To open it up and allow the person to talk about their feelings really *reduces* the risk. Negotiating, getting it out in the open, tends to bring in this sense of stability and consistency and honesty: 'We hear you, we're listening, we're trying to understand, we're trying to work together.'"

"As soon as you ask them, 'What are you doing?,'" agrees Dr. Tanney, "you're acknowledging their distress, you're valuing them as a person enough to listen to them and hear what they're saying – and you're offering, one assumes, to help them try to solve the problem so that they are no longer alone. And those are the four features that characterize suicide: you're alone, you don't see any other solutions to it, you don't value yourself very much, nobody cares about you."

One might assume that a person planning for suicide has already made an irrevocable decision to die – that your offer of assistance will not change things. In some cases that will be true. But in most, the ambivalence is a powerful tool to be worked with. The person will be grappling, painfully, between choosing life or death. The power of that ambivalence is dramatically illustrated by those who have attempted suicide and survived. Many people who have jumped from buildings or bridges remember thinking – as they plunged toward ground – "Wrong choice."

"A good number of them," explains Dr. Tanney, "clearly recall, on the way down, saying, 'You've done the wrong thing, you stupid idiot.' They do! So even after the event is in place, people are sort of going, 'I'm not sure whether I should have done it.'"

Twinned with ambivalence is the fact that the anguish of being acutely suicidal is too unbearable to last, in most cases, for extended periods. It is usually a *temporary* state of mind.

Which means that buying time, getting a person through a short but critical period, can be crucial.

Emphasize to the suicidal person that you will help them during this difficult phase. Reassure them it will not last forever – even though it may not feel that way. Offer realistic hope and avoid diminishing or belittling the pain they are suffering. Identify other supports, such as parents, friends, crisis lines, and professionals, and try to link the person to these helpers. If you believe the risk of suicide is immediate, don't leave them alone. A useful strategy can be to ask someone to *postpone* their decision regarding suicide. Even the most intense suicidal feelings, if they do not result in death, will lift.

"You're not necessarily waiting an entire week for that," says suicide researcher Ian Dawe. "It could just be waiting minutes to hours for that state of mind to change *enough* so that there's not going to be an attempt. There's an impulsive nature to the act. Anything that we can do to interrupt that impulse is a good thing. We see good results."

If you're doing the intervening, you may need help of your own. Share your concerns with someone you trust. Call your local crisis or suicide line; seek professional support. If you fear the person may harm themselves at any moment, further action may be warranted.

Hospitalization is one option. All provincial mental health laws permit involuntary hospitalization if a person is in danger of suicide. However, in cases where the person has had a previous, unpleasant experience in hospital, you may want to explore alternatives. Forcing someone in crisis to go somewhere against their will can add to their distress, though there are cases where this is appropriate.

"They may refuse adamantly to go to the hospital," points out Dr. Alain LeSage. "That may be understandable too, because it's a difficult place to be when you're on wards with people who are all, at least, very distressed."

A number of cities now offer non-hospital alternatives, including "safe houses" and crisis centres. Their atmosphere tends to be calmer than the hospital, the surroundings less clinical, the staff/client ratio higher. The vast majority include a medical component.

If it's felt the person is at imminent risk, try initially to provide them with a choice of places to go, based on local resources and their previous history. If the person is highly agitated and intent on death, hospitals are often the most appropriate place – especially if the individual has a trusted physician or therapist there.

"It's a safe place," adds Dr. LeSage. "You can provide twenty-four-hour supervision, very close supervision, when people are acutely suicidal."

When in doubt, have anyone who is suicidal assessed at the emergency ward of your local hospital – or by a mobile crisis team.

REMOVING THE MEANS

Another concrete step, when discussing suicide with someone at risk, is to ask them if they have a plan: if they have a *method* of suicide in mind. Research indicates that most people have a preferred way to die. If that particular method becomes unavailable – if the means of suicide is removed – they are less likely to consider alternative techniques.

Now couple that with some of the other key variables: the often impulsive nature of suicide, the ambivalence, the relatively short period in which people are most acutely suicidal. It adds up to another effective tool for intervention.

"Because the availability of means, plus the impulsivity, creates a sort of window of opportunity of despair," explains Dr. LeSage. "So, if during that period there's virtually no means, it might not happen. The danger zone may fade at that point."

"Suicide's a state of mind," emphasizes Dr. Links. "And if you don't have that gun there, or the bottle of Tylenol right in front of you, if you have to go that extra mile to get the means, it may be that the crisis passes and you come to decide that maybe there's another option here."

Obviously, one cannot eliminate every possible means of suicide from a home. But the removal of a gun or secure storage of medications or sharp knives – particularly if the person mentioned them as their plan – is a wise step. Your local police can assist in the removal and storage of any weapons.

THE YOUNG

Young people also see suicide as an option. Though Statistics Canada reported zero suicides in 1997 among children younger than ten, that picture changes as kids become young adults.

Number of Suicide Deaths by Age, 1997

	10–14 years	15–19 years
M	39	207
F	12	54

The rate of suicide rises dramatically for older adolescents. When expressed as a rate per 100,000 population of the fifteen to nineteen age group, this demographic shows the largest single increase of any category through life, jumping from a rate of 3.8 to 19.9 suicides. And the number of young people who ponder the act is staggering.

"You talk to kids," says Dr. Tanney, "and the data's pretty solid. Somewhere between 15% to 20% in a year think about killing themselves."

One of the largest studies of young people in Canada backs this up. The 1992 Adolescent Health Survey, conducted by the McCreary Centre Society in British Columbia, questioned 15,549 students from grades 7 through 12. It found that 16% reported considering suicide at least once during the preceding year, while 7% indicated they had actually attempted suicide during the same period.

In 1999, the Society released results of its Adolescent Health Survey II, which questioned 25,838 students. It found that while the number of young people who consider suicide had dropped to 14%, "a tragically high number of young people choose suicide as a response to difficult circumstances or personal despair."

So many that this country now has one of the highest rates of youth suicide in the industrialized world (a rate that has increased four-fold since the 1950s). In an article published in the October 1998 edition of the *Canadian Journal of Psychiatry*, Paul Links and colleague Anne Rhodes emphasized the stark trend.

"Post-World War II suicide rates have increased in youths," they wrote, "such that suicide is now the second leading cause of death in those under 45 years of age in Ontario. Studies indicate that 80% to 90% who die by suicide suffered from mental illness."

But what kinds of disorders?

"Depression, primarily, and other mood disorders," says Jennifer White, director of B.C.'s Suicide Prevention Information and Resource Centre. "Substance abuse is another key risk factor, as well as the experience of a recent loss. And so it's the combination of those things, not any one thing in isolation."

That recent loss – assuming the adolescent is already vulnerable – can be a small one. And White, who specializes in adolescent suicide, urges parents to understand that events which may seem insignificant to adults can be profound in the psyche of an at-risk teen.

"We have to be careful not to bring our adult lenses that have the benefit of lots of history and lots of experience," she cautions. "For young people [who are vulnerable] it can *feel* like the end of the world when they have a break-up of a relationship or they don't make a team, or they failed their driver's licence." White's statement echoes an observation made by Durkheim a hundred years ago: "We see some men resist horrible misfortune, while others kill themselves after slight troubles."

So what should a parent, relative, or teacher watch for? Pretty much the same things cited in the earlier list, along with unexpected drops in academic performance and withdrawal from relationships.

You can also keep an eye out for this:

"Kids who get very, very quiet," says Yvonne Bergmans, who has nearly two decades' experience working with high-risk groups, "and show real signs of anxiety or depression. Isolating themselves from their friends, believing that they can't, in fact, accomplish anything. There's this pervading sense of hopelessness."

A quiet, all-consuming hopelessness that runs far deeper and darker than mere teen angst; a sadness far more profound and prolonged than a case of the blues.

A number of recent works indicate that gay and lesbian youth may also be at increased risk. A 1999 Harvard study of 3,365 young people asked them whether they identified as being gay, lesbian, bisexual, or not sure of their sexual orientation. The survey also queried them about suicidal thoughts, plans, or attempts.

"Gay, lesbian, bisexual, or not sure youth," it concluded, "report a significantly increased frequency of suicide attempts."

Similar literature has been previously challenged, with critics questioning whether the surveys have indeed demonstrated a direct link. Perhaps the youngster made an attempt for reasons other than sexual orientation. Maybe there was dysfunction in the home, relationship troubles, problems at school. The last couple of years, however, have seen more pieces of peer-reviewed literature indicating that these youngsters *are* at increased risk, both of suicide and mental distress. Given the discrimination many gay and lesbian youth still endure, such data is not surprising.

Then there's the other type of young person. The driven perfectionist who seems to have everything together. The last person you'd suspect could be grappling with inner turmoil.

"They're excelling to a very high degree," says B.C.'s White, "and sometimes they get overlooked. But sometimes that kid, who suffers from such sensitivity to perceived criticism, can be the kind of kid who can also go on to die by suicide. It's the kid [about whom] I often hear people saying, 'Gee, I didn't see that coming.' But if you look back, you'll start to see that they had such impossibly high standards set for themselves that there was no room for mistake."

While there is no typical snapshot of a child at risk, it is clear that having a stable home life is a strong protective factor, that having an *un*stable home can drastically increase the vulnerability. "The single largest group [at risk]," says Dr. Tanney, "are clearly the disturbed adolescents who finally simply give up because of their turbulent family and developmental history."

Another risk factor, particularly during adolescence, is knowing someone else who has died of suicide. "Either a friend or family member," says clinical researcher Rahel Eynan. "That seems to be a risk factor." And it's a risk factor that can be compounded by media coverage that either romanticizes the tragedy or emphasizes the amount of grief it has caused. In several cases, a highly publicized youth suicide is thought to have triggered "suicide clusters" – a number of separate suicides that occur within a short time of the original death and which often use the same methods.

As with anyone suicidal, there's one signal that must not be ignored.

"The most obvious one," says Yvonne Bergmans, "is when a kid says, 'I wanna die.' And there are lots of kids who will say that." Those feelings might be expressed to a friend, sibling, parent – even a stranger. Some suicidal adolescents, perhaps more comfortable with the anonymity afforded by the Internet, will even post their thoughts online in search of support. The following passage was taken from a discussion group on suicide found at the Kid's Help Phone Internet site, <http://kidshelp.sympatico.ca/>.

Tequila – 04:47pm Oct 22
Guest User

*I'm not sure why I am writing this, but I am so depressed, I
hate my life, I have seriously considered suicide and I know that
no one would miss me in fact the world would be much better
off without me in the long run. I have never really been a happy
person, but I put on a great front, there are times when I break
down and let people see the real me but no one seems to care
when I do that so I don't anymore, I just feel like I am all alone
like there is no point anymore, I don't have any direction or
any motivation. I just feel so alone, I have sat with a whole
bunch of sleeping pills in my hand but then my sister came home
so I had to put them away. I guess I just don't know where I'm
headed or what I want and it is kind of scary.*

The pain, the ambivalence, the hopelessness are abundantly
clear in that single message. And it's important for the parent
or trusted figure to *accept* that the child really feels that way.

"People will say, 'You shouldn't feel like that,'" warns
Bergmans, "and disregard the full emotional reality that the kid
is living with." Such a response tends to diminish what the
adolescent is going through. The answer, as with anyone else,
is to listen, to offer support, to ask.

THE ELDERLY

Another group at risk of suicide is the elderly. In Canada, the
suicide rate for men spikes dramatically in the declining years.
Compare these numbers to the overall average rate of 19.6 suicides per 100,000 Canadian males:

Deaths per 100,000 Population, 1997 (Male)

65–69	70–74	75–79	80–84	85–89	90+
20.1	21.3	22.2	30.6	31.9	40.5

Unlike other age groups, the data indicates few of these people had any prior suicidal behaviour.

"When you look back in the elderly group who suicide," says Dr. Paul Links, "they often don't have the previous suicide attempts. So they may not have done this before, or indicated this kind of thought."

Suicide in the elderly is linked to risk factors that often include depression, physical pain, alcohol abuse, bereavement, loss of physical functions, and isolation. As with other suicide, rarely is it the result of a single crisis. Rather, it is generally a culmination of factors leading to overwhelming hopelessness and despair.

"And part of their hopelessness, their giving up on things," explains Dr. Links, "may be because they're now clinically depressed. So appropriate treatment seems to have a real important role in the elderly person at risk."

But Dr. Links stresses that in order to be appropriate, that treatment must take into account the combined factors which have led the person to become suicidal. Treating the depression alone reduces just a single risk factor, albeit a big one.

"We should be, hopefully, intervening across the spectrum," says Ian Dawe. "Whether that's the appropriate treatment of a depression, whether it's the control of the physical ailments, whether it's the social isolation. Hopefully it's all three of those things that are manageable. And that's really going to make an effective difference."

A reference guide published by the Suicide Information and Education Centre in Calgary (SIEC) (<http://www.siec.ca>) concurs that there are several strategies which can reduce the incidence of elderly suicide. In addition to conventional treatment, the SIEC recommends support in the areas of housing, income, and retirement preparation.

It also points out an oft-neglected approach that can bring renewed meaning to the life of someone at risk: "Recognition of the value of elderly persons and greater respect for their experience and knowledge."

THE AFTERMATH

Unfortunately, suicide is unpredictable. Not everyone will send overt signals that they are considering ending their life. Not everyone will ask for help; not everyone will accept it. Some people, despite our very best efforts, will die. And the act leaves tremendous trauma in its wake.

"Although the numbers of deaths and years of lost life can be counted," reads the 1994 Task Force Report, "it is impossible to assess the waste of economic potential for Canada and the legacy of human misery that suicides leave behind to surviving family and friends." By one estimate, six other people are directly, often profoundly, affected by every single suicide.

"And this is *direct* impact," explains Dr. Links. "Quite directly their life and functioning is affected. And the impact of suicide is probably more significant than any other death."

Why?

"It leaves a person probably with more guilt than any other death."

So much guilt and pain, that those who've lost someone to suicide are themselves subsequently at higher risk of ending their lives. And *that* risk is frequently exacerbated by the reluctance of friends, family – of society in general – to discuss suicide openly and directly. Professionals emphasize the importance of "post-vention" – dealing with the grief, anger, or self-blame in the wake of a suicide death.

Support groups for those bereft by suicide exist in many Canadian cities. One of the largest, the Survivor Support Program, is based in Toronto. During its twenty-two years in existence, the program has helped more than ten thousand people cope. Executive director Karen Letofsky says the taboos surrounding suicide can rob survivors of important support.

"Whether it's the reluctance of the individual bereft by suicide to reach out to friends," she says, "or the reluctance of friends to want to discuss the topic – either way it leads to social isolation."

Doris Sommer-Rotenberg, whose son Arthur ended his life at the age of thirty-six, still recalls the intense regret she felt; the helpless, futile pain.

"There's a guilt in every death, there's no question," she says. "You think of all the things that you should have done, or didn't do, or whatever. But I think with suicide everyone feels it even more. Certainly I do."

Arthur Sommer-Rotenberg was in the depths of depression when he killed himself. A successful doctor, highly intelligent and outgoing, Arthur had been diagnosed with bipolar affective disorder when he was seventeen. He'd endured four episodes, the harsh swings between the electric highs and the crushing lows.

Not long before his death, he came to visit his mother. Doris Sommer-Rotenberg was busy at a meeting. Arthur told her he was going upstairs to lie down, as he'd done on other occasions when depressed, but left the house shortly afterward. It was the last time she saw him alive. One week later, his grieving mother was left, as are many bereft by suicide, wondering if she could have done something differently.

"The listening is extremely important," she reflects. "And that's the one tremendous regret I have with Arthur: that I was always trying to fix it instead of just listen. I only had the most awful sense that I wished I could have taken him in my arms and could have somehow given him the comfort and the desire to go on."

Some friends were incredibly supportive following her son's death. Others shunned her. Suicide was just too difficult for many to acknowledge. "They feel it's contagious," she recalls, "they don't want to be contaminated, they won't have anything to do with you."

But Doris Sommer-Rotenberg, despite her anguish, was determined not to let her son's death overshadow his life. She immediately began a campaign to create an academic suicide research program – one she would name in her son's honour.

The result of Doris's efforts is the Arthur Sommer Rotenberg Chair in Suicide Studies. It is, first and foremost, a lasting memorial to her son – recognition of a wonderful life. And it is an appropriate tribute, given his passion for medicine. As much as anything, however, establishing the program was an empowering and positive way for Doris to cope with her son's death.

"Setting up the chair was extraordinarily helpful to me," she explains, "because I wasn't just sitting there grieving and absorbing all the pain inside. I was able, in a sense, to transmute the tragedy into something that gave his life meaning and gave his death meaning. And that helped me tremendously.

"Though I will never recover from Arthur's death, as a friend recently said, neither did I become entrapped by it."

A large graduation photo of Arthur hangs proudly at the program's headquarters; a separate photo album celebrates his adventurous life, his love of travel. Virtually every picture is dominated by his infectious, exuberant smile.

NOMI'S STORY *

Healing is a matter of time. But how does one measure it? In days? In months? In years? Is sooner better than later? Is there such a thing as too little time? Or even too much?

Unfortunately, healing is a process without maps or guidelines. It's as individual as the wounds we suffer. Mine was the suicide of my nineteen-year-old brother, Peter, in 1968.

Confronted with the choice of living with the trauma of his death and going mad, or burying it and going on, I chose to bury it. And for the next twenty-seven years, it stayed buried, while I remained frozen in the grief process.

But if grief was my prison, guilt was its warden. Because my brother's last words to me were, "Help me." Three weeks later he was dead. And I was left haunted. Haunted by my failure as a sister to save her only sibling's life. Haunted, too, by anger and denial. Sadness and loss. And pain. Violent, searing pain.

Whenever I looked for the answer as to why my brother died, I was told, "Hey, it was the Sixties." To blame the times

* This story was originally published in a slightly different form in *Open Minds*, a newsletter produced by the Writer's Circle, in Sudbury, Ontario. The project encourages consumer/survivors to write for pleasure, publication, or both. Reprinted by permission.

for his destruction seemed logical enough. For if ever anyone defined the Sixties, it was my brother. Brilliant. Inquisitive. Adventurous. Fearless.

A marginal student, he dropped out of university to live with friends as part of Montreal's hippie community. And it was in that netherworld of drugs and pseudo-Eastern philosophies that he rose, quickly and briefly, to prominence.

In a desperate bid to save his life, my parents signed the papers committing him to the Douglas Hospital for observation and treatment. Two days before his scheduled commitment, he was arrested by the RCMP and jailed. My father, an attorney, had him released on bail to enter hospital, but he was discharged – without my parents' consent – after a mere twelve-day stay. Six days later, he was dead.

That night, I wrote the first in a series of poems about him. It was to be my only form of consolation from then on. And so, whenever I felt that familiar surge of pain inside me, I'd write a poem. Then I'd slip it into the large plastic box that lay hidden at the back of my clothes closet. As time passed, I found other, more public outlets for my pain: short stories and eventually novels. Seven of them in eleven years.

But where my professional life flourished, my personal life floundered. After my brother's death, I stopped using his name. To me, it was tantamount to sacrilege. Like taking the name of the Lord in vain. And I stopped talking about him. To my parents, my husband, my friends.

Of the two of us, I'd always considered myself the weaker one, the overly sensitive one, the depressed one. If anyone were likely to commit suicide, it would have been me. Once I even told my parents, "His death has sentenced me to life."

Because I was the only child left, I took it upon myself to be both daughter and son to my parents. I needed to make up to them for what my brother had done. But I also felt the need to apologize for being the one left behind.

Always fearful, I grew increasingly so over the years. I sought help from several therapists, yet we touched only briefly on my brother. Whenever we did, I considered the matter dealt with and closed. I thought I was fine, that I was getting on well with my life. But I was wrong. We still had unfinished business, my brother and I.

Then, in 1995, I suddenly became obsessed with the need to know the truth – not only about my brother's death, but about his life as well. And so I set aside my fiction and embarked on what proved to be a journey, both of discovery and self-discovery, culminating in the publication of my book My Brother Peter.

During my intensive search, I learned, among other things, that my brother had been well-loved. That everyone who'd known him had thought him extraordinary. They talked to me about his unique intelligence. His boundless energy and creativity. His charm. His generosity. His magnetic personality. Said one of his friends, "Peter didn't pass through people's lives unnoticed. Those who experienced him are still holding pieces of him."

What a tribute to him. What a comfort to me. I hoarded each precious accolade like a miser hoarding priceless gems, and used them as paving stones for my path to healing.

But I wasn't alone on that path. With me was my long-time therapist, who helped me do what I'd never been able to do before: strip away the armour that had shielded my heart for so long. He taught me that the more one talks about a painful subject, the less power that subject has. The more one's exposed to a particular trauma, the less frightening that trauma becomes.

And so, I began to talk. And as I talked, we began to separate the strands of emotions, starting with my anger. I learned that I'd halted its natural evolution in order to protect myself. To heal, I would have to direct my anger at its rightful target: at my brother, for squandering his potential and throwing away his life.

I learned that by stopping the grief process, I was preserving my brother as the brother I remembered: kind and good, funny and sweet, loyal and loving. That way I wouldn't have to admit that the young man I'd adored, who, with his near-genius IQ, could have been anything and done anything, had chosen instead to drop out of society and deal in drugs.

And I learned that my guilt was misplaced. I could not have saved him. By the end, the sheer quantity of marijuana and LSD he'd ingested would have changed him utterly and completely. The choice he made to end his life would have been the choice of a mind destroyed by the very drugs he'd originally used to expand that mind.

After many, many months of talking, I finally asked my therapist about closure. He told me that it, too, was an evolutionary process. And that I'd know I'd achieved it when I had a feeling of release, a feeling of peacefulness.

Thankfully, I have both of those feelings now. Because I have, finally, begun to heal. The grief has faded. The guilt has eased. The anger has lessened. And the pain has been reduced to a tender, bittersweet ache. The sadness, though, remains. Because to put it simply: I miss him. Miss what he might have been. Miss what we might have shared together. His dying tore a jagged hole in my psyche, and although I've stopped expecting it to close completely, it has begun to shrink, and the edges are smoother now.

I've travelled a great distance since the start of my journey, and learned more than I'd ever expected to learn. To me, however, the greatest lesson has been this: there can be an end to the grief process; one can seek and ultimately find peace of mind. No matter how late one starts down the path to healing, it is never, never too late.

I draw my strength from that and carry on.

CHAPTER ELEVEN

Stigma

"We're outcasts. We're 'untouchables.'" – *John*

John has a diagnosis of schizophrenia. And for him, that label – people's *reaction* to that label – has been an albatross. Never mind that he's happily married, that he's funny, that he knows hockey inside out. Doesn't matter. He's been crazy. Therefore, he's somehow "not one of us." Not normal. Less than normal. *Abnormal.*

The word "stigma" is Greek in origin – and its meaning had nothing to do with mental health. It referred to the practice of burning or cutting a mark into the flesh of criminals and slaves. The mark served to make their status apparent to all; a label that would set them permanently apart.

In some ways, we haven't made much progress. We still brand people. The physical markings may be gone, but an invisible stamp of "the other" is often squarely applied to the forehead of someone with a mental disorder. It remains *the* most common concern voiced by consumers.

"Stigma," goes an oft-repeated saying, "is worse than the disorder."

Unless you've been on the receiving end, it's tough to comprehend how that statement could possibly be true. Surely the *disorder* is the problem – and once that's under control everything else is fine, right? Well, in a perfect world that would be the case. People with mental health problems would be universally regarded as equal members of society. They would be supported by understanding co-workers, landlords, friends, and family. They would be seen for who they are – not what they've been diagnosed with.

Unfortunately, the real world doesn't work that way. While there's been some progress, having a mental disorder can still throw up roadblocks to friendship, housing, and work.

"You should call stigma what it is," one woman stated bluntly: "Discrimination."

The kind of discrimination where a Canadian bank can refuse loan insurance if you've ever been diagnosed with a mental disorder. Where private health insurance can be denied if you've ever seen a psychiatrist. Where a Canadian diagnosed with a major mental disorder can be denied entry to the United States. Discrimination based on fear, misunderstanding, and just plain ignorance. A mindset that excludes rather than includes. More than one person has compared it to apartheid.

Such an extreme comparison may not be too far off. Perhaps the starkest example of prejudice we've noticed was on the manicured grounds of a major psychiatric hospital in Toronto. Just a few metres from a busy sidewalk was a simple sign. It was supposed to read: "Dogs must be kept on a leash." Except someone had crossed out the first word and replaced it with something else.

"Nuts must be kept on a leash."

That sign remained untouched for eight months, until someone sprayed black paint over the offending word.

Now imagine a slightly different scenario. Picture a similar sign on the grounds of a synagogue. If the word "dogs" had been replaced by "Jews," people would have been outraged. The police would likely have been called. The act would have been described, accurately, as a hate crime. And, rest assured, the sign would have been replaced immediately.

All winter, that sign at the hospital remained unaltered. It would have been impossible for staff to miss it. It would have been impossible for patients to miss it. It would have been impossible for the public to miss it. And yet no one did a thing.

That isn't the only sign of prejudice floating around. In a 1998 edition of a Toronto tabloid newspaper, there was a story about the Capitol Hill shootings in Washington, D.C., an act committed by a man with schizophrenia. The headline read: "No Hiding from Nutters." Imagine the outcry had a different "N" word had been used.

A national business magazine ran an ad for a clothing chain featuring a man in a straitjacket. His eyes were bulging, his hair unkempt. He looked, in a Three Stooges kind of way, absolutely and utterly "mad." Though the intent was humorous, those who've been in restraints found nothing to laugh about.

A Saskatchewan radio station used to proudly bill its morning crew as the "psycho club." A major Toronto station, during its newscast, reported that Margaret Trudeau Kemper, former wife of Pierre Trudeau, was being held in "the nuthouse." The Jim Carrey movie *Me, Myself & Irene* was promoted with the slogan: "From Gentle to Mental." Entertainment reporters were given press kits with candy "pills" that were jokingly packaged as a "cure" for schizophrenia.

The list goes on. And on.

In isolation, those examples may not appear significant to some readers (which, in itself, is a statement of the pervasiveness of stigma). Together, however, they reflect – and reinforce – an implicit societal belief. It's okay to treat these people differently. Okay, because they *are* different. As a document published by the World Federation for Mental Health points out, misconceptions still abound.

"Those with mental illnesses, some would say, are getting what they deserve as a result of their own personal inadequacies," it states. "They are perceived, for example, as lacking the motivational resolve to overcome their problems, as lazy, as self-indulgent in their emotions; they have simply given in to stress and failed to pull themselves up by their bootstraps as would a person of stronger character."

Those words echo the findings of the CMHA's Ontario Division. In 1993–94, it contracted an outside firm to assist in developing an anti-stigma campaign. As part of its research, the firm surveyed people working in the mental health field for their opinions on which attitudinal barriers were most pervasive. The respondents, by percentage, stated that the following beliefs are most prevalent. That people with a mental illness:

are dangerous or violent	88%
lack intelligence or are developmentally handicapped	40%
cannot function/cannot hold a job/have nothing to contribute	32%
lack willpower/are weak or lazy	24%
are unpredictable/can't be trusted	20%
are to blame/should shape up	20%

The research also revealed that social and family life, along with employment, were the areas most frequently identified as being negatively affected by stigma. High percentages of respondents said stigma impaired:

social and family relationships	84%
employment	78%
housing	48%
inclusion in the community	22%
self-esteem	20%

Is that *really* possible? Could stigma truly affect so many aspects of a person's life? Meet Harold, a middle-aged man with a diagnosis of bipolar affective disorder.

His story begins well enough. Harold had fallen in love. It was the most wonderful thing that had happened to him – and his self-esteem – in years. Wonderful, too, because the object of his affection didn't care about his diagnosis. She loved Harold for who he was.

Assuming her parents would share her excitement, she told them all about the man in her life – including his diagnosis. But that last bit was a mistake.

"Her parents don't want her to go out with me because I'm a manic-depressive," Harold says, adding bitterly, "even though they've never met me."

For Harold, it was a stark reminder of the many other doors stigma has slammed. Doors he desperately wanted to be open. He has learned, the hard way, that there can be times when honesty is not the best policy.

"If I tell a prospective employer about my illness, they just won't give me a job," he says. "They don't say so directly, but I can tell from their facial expressions and the questions they ask me. I tried being honest about it, but found I'm better off not mentioning it."

Because Harold can't find a permanent job, he doesn't have a lot of money.

"As a result I can't afford to eat properly, and I can't go out on dates or be supportive financially in a normal relationship. I just can't do it, and it's very frustrating."

Harold's story shows, dramatically, how detrimental stigma can be. It has affected his relationship, his employment prospects, his income. And those setbacks have all had a direct impact on his mental health. Some consumer/survivors refer to stigma as "crazy-making," meaning it can really do a number on your head.

Stories like Harold's are all too common. A major U.S. study released in 1997 by the National Alliance for the Mentally Ill (NAMI) surveyed 1,388 people diagnosed with schizophrenia, bipolar affective disorder, and major depression. The work was conducted by Otto Wahl, a clinical psychologist widely known for his scientific research on the impact of stigma.

The study revealed that one in three respondents had been turned down for a job for which they were qualified because of a psychiatric diagnosis. Fully seven out of ten said they'd been treated as less competent in the workplace when their diagnosis was revealed.

"When I was first diagnosed," one person told the study, "I made the mistake of telling my supervisor at the time what was going on. She decided I couldn't have a job I'd been doing for ten years and demoted me."

"I only reveal that I am a consumer to people I know very well," wrote another respondent. "Nor do I reveal it in any situation when that could hurt me, such as applying for a job. I simply lie. I do not give them a chance to hurt me with their misunderstanding."

And such misunderstandings *do* hurt. Consider this Quebec woman's story, which first appeared (along with others quoted here) in the *Toronto Star* series "Out of Mind."

My name is Catherine and I am from Montreal. In 1994 I had a big psychosis and was hospitalized for 6 weeks. Though my breakdown did not occur at work, I was very open and told my co-workers what happened to me. Since then they do not treat me the same way. First of all, they believe that I am not capable of handling stress, so they believe that I am not capable of handling certain tasks. Also, I have overheard one of my co-workers tell a new employee that I had gone wacko. I work part-time now and people think that I am just lazy and that I go home early to watch soap operas. I find myself in the situation that I must find myself another job where nobody knows my past, so that I can be treated like a normal human being again.

Catherine's experience touches on a number of important issues. The first is that she wanted to be able to tell her co-workers what had happened to her. Having a psychotic episode and being hospitalized are major events in anyone's life – especially if they've happened for the first time. There can be a tremendous desire to explain what happened to friends or colleagues, to have them somehow understand what you've gone through. The one thing Catherine needed more than anything was the one thing she was denied – understanding.

She was also subjected to what might be referred to as lowered expectations. While it's true that less stressful environments can be helpful for some people, it is often assumed that anyone with a mental health issue is now incapable of performing tasks they used to handle routinely. Catherine's frustration with this is clear. Add on the water-cooler gossip, and this woman, understandably, is now looking for work elsewhere.

Deciding whether to tell co-workers about a disorder is a very personal choice. While the office can be a cruel environment, we know of other consumers who've been treated sensitively, supportively, and fairly. Responses seem to vary according to the nature and severity of the disorder (schizophrenia tends to be more stigmatized than anxiety), and the progressiveness of the workplace. A good rule of thumb, *if* you wish to disclose, is to tell only those colleagues who have become good and trusted friends – and tell them outside of the workplace. Only you can decide if it's necessary – or desirable – to tell your employer.

Misconceptions are so widespread, however, that you can feel stigmatized even when others *don't know* you have a mental disorder. This next story illustrates how one man felt untouched by stigma – until he really started to think about it.

I am 38 years old and had my first break [schizophrenia] at the age of 30. I have not had any stigma heaped on me personally, but I do have to sit and listen to co-workers sometimes as they describe the people across the street. You see, where I work is across the street from a psychiatric hospital (one in which I have never set foot) and almost every day someone says something about the people that come and go from there. I have heard someone say, as if it were fact, that all people with mental illness chose to be that way, that they had simply given up on things and needed a swift boot in the butt to get better. I just sit and listen a lot of times, other times I may say something about how ill-informed they are. I don't

do that too often as I do not want to give myself away. I am
fortunate that no one can tell I have a problem just by looking
at me. Now that I come to think of it, perhaps stigma does
affect me after all or otherwise I would tell people what is
wrong with me.

Stigma, then, can be surreptitious; you don't have to be
the direct target to feel its sting. The story also conveys the
fact that stigma *pre*-judges; the comments about the psychiatric patients were made by people who knew nothing about
them as individuals. (Just as Harold had never met his girlfriend's parents, just as the employers in Otto Wahl's study
never gave the job applicants a chance.)

That is perhaps the most devastating aspect of stigma: the
misconceptions are *automatically* applied, denying the person
any opportunity to disprove them. When that happens to a
person again and again, it's not unusual for them to internal-
ize that stigma and start losing hope.

And when hope diminishes, so do the odds of returning to
sound mental health. This unfortunate fact is highlighted on
the first page of a global anti-stigma program sponsored
by the World Psychiatric Association (WPA). Although the
Open the Doors program is specifically aimed at the stigma
and discrimination associated with schizophrenia, the impact
can be felt by anyone with a serious mental disorder.

"Stigma can become the main cause for social isolation,
inability to find work, alcohol and drug abuse, homelessness,
and excessive institutionalization," reads the report, "all of
which decrease the chance of recovery."

Think about that for a minute. Imagine what it would be
like to have no friends, no chance of finding work. Visualize
how it might feel to be marginalized, disenfranchised, scraping by on a disability pension. Try to conceive of a community
so stigmatizing that even your children are picked on.

Then read the story of this woman, who wrote to us from
the U.S. We've heard near-identical stories from many
Canadians.

I am a 44-year-old, with children.

I was diagnosed 6 yrs ago as schizo-affective. It's still an uphill battle.

I live in a very small town.

There was no way to keep my illness a secret.

I am rarely taken seriously by the townspeople. You see, I'm "mad."

I am either dismissed or ignored. I have no friends.

I am, as of yet, unable to work. The doctors are still trying to find the right meds for me. I've been on disability for 4 yrs. If it weren't for the kindness of my ex-husband and my mother . . . there is no way we could have made it to where we are now. Public assistance cannot support a family. It is definitely inadequate to properly care for children. Between my schizophrenia and our low income my children were exposed to the worst treatment. They are singled out for a lot of cruelty. They have few friends and little hope for the future. They are even having trouble finding employment, due to stigma. You see, their father also had the disorder. So they are also burdened with the possibility of having the disorder themselves. I am blessed and thank God that their reaction has been to "bury" themselves in their studies. Just the thought of the alternatives makes me shudder.

The stigma must end. The children, the future, is at stake.

It is little wonder this woman remains unwell – and little surprise that, after six years of trying, her doctors haven't been able to find the right medications. Pills will not correct her neighbours' attitudes.

Some of the scientific literature suggests this woman might be better off elsewhere – such as on the other side of the world. The WPA's anti-stigma campaign cites studies showing that the course of schizophrenia tends to be more benign, with fewer and shorter psychotic breaks, in developing nations.

"The reason for the better outcome in the developing world is not completely understood," says the report, "but it may be due to the fact that many people with mental illness in villages in the developing world are better accepted, less stig-matised, and more likely to find work in the subsistence agricultural economy. . . .

"Another striking difference is that, in developing countries, individuals with schizophrenia are more likely to remain in the community with their families, which helps protect them from becoming socially isolated and perhaps leads to a better prog-nosis. This theory is supported by research indicating that social isolation is associated with a worse outcome in schizophrenia."

THE SOURCES OF STIGMA

Who, as a child, hasn't called someone a "psycho" or a "schiz?" What campfire would be complete without a story about the axe-wielding lunatic who escaped from the nearby "funny farm"? How many movies have you seen where the villain was not merely bad, but mad?

Stigma has, in many respects, long been part of our culture; an insular, secure world where anything remotely beyond the confines of "normal" can inspire derision, fear, or both. Think of the homophobic AIDS jokes that went around in the 1980s. The not-so-discrete stares people still direct toward those with physical limitations or facial anomalies. The schoolyard chants that continue to ridicule the weak, the geek, the fat, the freak. It seems to be part of our nature to separate "us" from "them."

We've done this on a vast scale with the mentally unwell. Few human conditions have merited such widespread and enduring segregation; much of our treatment this century has been akin to quarantine. Our approach, until a few short decades ago, was to care for people in psychiatric institutions hidden from the rest of the world. Although the intentions may have been hon-ourable, the signal to the public at large was that these folks were clearly very different from "us." A people apart.

It's a perception the media have done little to counter. Hollywood loves its psycho killers, as does prime time. Content analysis of American television has shown that a staggering 72% of fictional characters with mental disorders are portrayed as violent. Similar studies of newspapers in Canada and Britain have shown that stories about violent acts involving the mentally disordered appear more frequently, are longer, and are more likely to receive prominent placement than stories with a positive or sympathetic message.

That would be justifiable, were there a clear and strong correlation between mental disorder and violence. But there is not.

"There's no question that some of the violence in society can be attributed to [serious] mental disorder," says prominent U.S. researcher Dr. John Monahan, who specializes in the topic. "The best estimates are that it's in the neighbourhood of 4%. So that even if mental disorder could be magically cured tomorrow, 96% of violence in society would still be there."

Dr. Julio Arboleda-Flórez, head of the department of psychiatry at Queen's University, thinks even the estimate of 4% may be high. Were you to attempt to determine the contribution mental disorder makes to societal violence as a whole, he says, "then it's so small that it's difficult to measure."

(The debate over violence and mental disorder is a complicated one, and designing studies to measure any relationship accurately is fraught with difficulty. But few would argue with the fact that the media grossly overemphasizes any connection. You can find an in-depth article Scott wrote on the topic at <http://atkinsonfdn.on.ca>.)

This problem with presenting a skewed or biased portrait is all the more disturbing when you consider the media's power, both to inform and misinform.

In recent years, advocates, reporters, and responsible editors have made efforts to get more representative stories published or broadcast. But it only takes a high-profile negative story or two before they're back to square one. The World Psychiatric Association recently discovered this in Alberta.

In co-operation with the WPA's campaign, the *Calgary Herald* supported placing more favourable, explanatory coverage about schizophrenia into the newspaper. Dr. Arboleda-Flórez, who was involved in the project, watched as the number of positive stories rose by an average 35%

throughout a sixteen-month period. The paper also devoted more space than usual to these non-stigmatizing stories, boosting their length by 16%. Progress, right?

Then in the U.S. came the Unabomber arrest and a shooting on Capitol Hill, and in Canada a subway pushing in Toronto – a string of high-profile cases involving men with diagnoses of schizophrenia. Those stories, with the Unabomber leading the charge, helped fuel a 44% increase in what was deemed "negative" coverage of schizophrenia during the same period.

"Obviously," says Arboleda-Flórez, "every time a case of this nature takes place, then the stigma goes up immediately."

Arboleda-Flórez has published previously on the Canadian media and stigma; he's also done extensive work on dangerousness. He notes that reporters and editors automatically assume that the disorder was directly responsible for the crime. "The newspaper usually says, 'The person was known to have a mental illness,'" he observes, "or, 'The person was not on treatment.' And that increases the perception in the public: 'Oooh – mental patients do these crazy things.' Yeah. But how many times do we have a person who is *not* mentally ill doing some serious crime in the community? And does he get the same perception in the public?"

The factors that contribute to stigma are myriad. But it's worth touching on one more – an ironic twist that can turn into a downward spiral of prejudice and isolation. And that is when the treatment itself marks the person.

As noted in Chapter 8, a fair proportion of people who've been on certain antipsychotic medications develop unwanted movement disorders over time. Involuntary grimaces, pacing, shuffling, or tremors can become quite apparent.

It is these drug side effects – the smacking of lips, the rocking, the restlessness – that fit our stereotypes of "crazy" behaviour. Few members of the public realize that these odd tics are induced by medication, as opposed to being symptoms of "madness." As the WPA anti-stigma program notes:

"The treatments patients receive may also increase the stigma associated with the illness. Especially if they produce the debilitating motor side effects that can result from treatment with certain antipsychotic medications."

Enough bad news. Time for something positive.

FIGHTING BACK

While there is still much to be done, there has been progress. People with an interest in mental health are now far more likely to challenge stigmatizing or inaccurate portrayals – often with very successful results. Quite often, too, these advocates discover there was no malice on the part of those responsible for the stigma; the perpetrators were merely misinformed or had no idea how sensitive the issue was.

In the United States, a group called Stigmabusters is a leading watchdog. But there are also significant efforts underway in this country. The CMHA, with its Open Mind campaign, has been working to sensitize the media, contacting journalists directly when stigmatizing articles appear. The Schizophrenia Society has worked long and hard to debunk some of the pervasive myths surrounding the disorder. And many individual consumer/survivors, by telling their stories and speaking publicly, have been chipping away at those walls.

The newly formed Canadian Alliance for Mental Illness and Mental Health (CAMIMH) promises to place stigma at the top of its agenda. There has been talk of a national anti-stigma campaign, and this group has the clout to achieve it. The alliance includes all the major players in Canada: the Canadian Psychiatric Association, the CMHA, the Mood Disorders Association, the Schizophrenia Society, and the consumer/ survivor group National Network for Mental Health.

Their work could achieve real results, because it's been shown that mindsets *can* be changed. The World Psychiatric Association's anti-stigma campaign in Alberta, for example, used a wide range of educational activities. Consumer/survivors spoke at schools, informative radio ads were played, humanizing pamphlets and posters distributed. Telephone surveys of eight hundred people conducted before and after the campaign showed a significant reduction in stigmatizing attitudes toward schizophrenia and the people who live with it.

It's worth pointing out that fighting stigma is also an empowering process for those who've endured it. Many consumer/survivors report feeling better about themselves as a result of taking some sort of action.

Here's how you can help.

- Join one of the organizations listed above. The greater the membership in these groups, the greater their political clout. (Although don't try to join the CPA unless you're a psychiatrist!)
- Voice your opinion. Write to media organizations that perpetuate myths about mental health. Even today, some reporters still think schizophrenia is "split personality." Politely critique any inaccuracies with a constructive tone, possibly including some pamphlets on mental disorder. Copy your letter to the managing editor.
- Contact advertisers or manufacturers that send stigmatizing messages. Let them know that not only are they offending you – they're likely offending some 20% of their potential customers. Remember, one in five people will experience a diagnosable mental disorder in any given year.
- Take part in campaigns like Open Mind or other stigma-fighting efforts. It's a great way to meet people and achieve something positive. If your local self-help group isn't doing anything, consider organizing interested consumer/survivors.
- When you hear someone make an offensive or insensitive remark concerning mental disorder, let them know it's not amusing. Anyone concerned about stigma can do this – you don't have to be a consumer/survivor.
- If you can document that you've been discriminated against because of mental disorder – and if you feel strong

enough – consider taking your case to a provincial human-rights organization or the Canadian Human Rights Commission.

- Use "People First" language. Avoid such dehumanizing terms as "a schizophrenic" when talking about a person diagnosed with schizophrenia. We don't refer to a person with cancer as "a canceric."
- Be human. When you see someone on the street apparently suffering from a mental disorder, don't veer away. A polite smile or nod – an acknowledgement they exist – will be valued.
- Be open about mental disorder. Being shameful, or feeling like you have to hide it, is a victory for stigma. The more these issues are talked about, the more accepted they'll become.

"People need to talk about it," says former federal finance minister Michael Wilson. "The fundamental [problem] is that people do not view mental illness the same way as a broken leg, or an ulcer, or cancer, or AIDS. People who have mental illness – depression, schizophrenia, whatever it is – you [shouldn't] write them off."

These may appear to be small steps. But each one is a step *forward* in a struggle that will eventually be won.

A PERSONAL NOTE FROM SCOTT

Stigma was, for me, the most agonizing aspect of my disorder. It cost friendships, career opportunities, and – most importantly – my self-esteem. It wasn't long before I began *internalizing* the attitudes of others, viewing myself as a lesser person.

In fact, this process began the moment I received a diagnosis. Like many consumer/survivors, I had my own baggage, my own preconceptions of what having a mental disorder meant. And so the stigma I had unknowingly carried toward others was turned inward. Many of those long days in bed during the depression were spent thinking, "I'm mentally ill. I'm a manic-depressive. I'm not the *same* anymore." I wondered, desperately, if I would ever again work, ever again be "normal." It was a godawful feeling that contributed immensely to the suicidal yearnings that invaded my thoughts.

When the depression finally lifted, I thought I'd survived everything. But being back on the job brought its own moments of purgatory. There is a uniquely penetrating type of pain that comes with silence, stares, awkwardness. The fears I'd conquered, the obstacles I'd overcome, began resurfacing all at once. Over time, I started thinking those people who avoided me in the halls might be right. Perhaps I was now less than I had been. After all, I'd gone crazy. Maybe I even *looked* "mentally ill."

But not everyone reacted like that. A few friends and co-workers did something so simple it was extraordinary. They ignored the brand. They still wanted to work together on a story, see a movie, go fishing – hang out. They still saw *me*.

And because they still saw me, I began wondering what it was all those other people were looking at.

One day, I figured it out. I finally understood what they were seeing. A myth.

And that realization was the best of all. Because stigma wasn't my problem any more.

It was theirs.

JULIE'S STORY *

It's hard to describe what it is like to live with a person who has a mental illness. It's even harder to explain the sadness, as a parent, to watch this disease rob your child of normalcy. And it borders on ridiculous, how victims and their families are treated when a mental diagnosis has been given.

Reaching a diagnosis for a mentally ill child is an epic and very frustrating journey. Often, children's symptoms do not mirror standard adult criteria, and even more often, parents feel responsible for bizarre and uncontrollable behaviours. And sadly, parents are blamed, even when a disorder is diagnosed, as being bad, defective, abusive, and/or deficient.

My fifteen-year-old daughter, Helen, suffers from bipolar disorder, social phobic disorder, and is also phobic to water, needles, and pain in general. The combination of disorders is difficult to medicate properly, and is a constant challenge. When Helen is manic, her phobias disappear. Mood stabilizers bring phobias back with a vengeance. Antidepressants (Prozac, Zoloft, and

---

* This story was originally published in a slightly different form in *Open Minds*, a newsletter produced by the Writer's Circle, in Sudbury, Ontario. The project encourages consumer/survivors to write for pleasure, publication, or both. Reprinted by permission.

310

Paxil) only cause a multitude of bipolar symptoms to return. Wellbutrin, with Helen, caused severe facial tics.

The mood stabilizers we've tried are Depakote, Tegretol, Lithobid, and Eskalith, which Helen currently takes. Even on mood stabilizers, Helen still experiences mild manic and severe depressive episodes. Stress and hormonal fluctuations seem to bring on these episodes and have kept us from medicinal success for the last three years.

The most frightening aspect of Helen's illnesses is the threat of fatality. During the summer of 1997, she attempted suicide through overdose. We knew Helen had suicidal ideas, and I had read about the high incidence of suicide, but I never thought we would see her attempt it. She always assured us she would never try to take her life. I don't take this aspect lightly any longer.

If Helen's illnesses were our only struggles, it would be more than enough for any family. Unfortunately, there are bigger demons than mental illness to live with. Prejudice and stigma take on a life of their own. Not only do you watch your child suffer, you are isolated and left with no support or sympathy. You fight for respect and acceptance from family, friends, and schools. It's exhausting, and it comes as no surprise to me that so many victims and their families live quietly in shame, guilt, and embarrassment.

Our school district has repeatedly told me that simply having a mental illness does not afford a child the right to special services. There is nothing simple about mental illness. Our schools should be required to provide specialized services for all children diagnosed with mental disorders. We cannot continue to allow the mentally ill to be held responsible for an illness they are unable to control. We must give them acceptance, room to acquire skills, and appropriate education.

The most hurtful prejudice has come from the people I thought I could depend on in times of crisis. I have a few supportive friends and my loving mother, but my entire large family is ashamed and intolerant of Helen, her illnesses, and associated symptoms. We aren't invited to family gatherings, holiday meals, or celebrations. I wish I were a bigger and better person, but I must admit that I am very bitter. However, I don't feel that our *loss was great. If I had to choose between Helen and my family, Helen would win hands down!*

I have no sage advice regarding the prejudice directed towards the mentally ill. It is truly worse than the illness itself. My choice has been not to hide, be embarrassed, or accept any shame or guilt. We speak openly of Helen's illnesses, and those who cannot handle it are not part of our life. I feel this is the only way to give Helen self-respect, and the only way to gradually eradicate prejudice.

Living with Helen has taught me that mental illness is not a weakness of character, but rather a disease that requires the strongest of character.

CHAPTER TWELVE

A Home, a Job, a Friend

As Julia and I complete this project, our two offices are overflowing with notebooks, studies, policy manuals, interview transcripts, books. There are many tens of thousands of pages crammed into these tiny rooms – everything from the official Australian mental health policy to a Canadian book condemning electroconvulsive therapy. It is a diverse collection of science, politics, human experience. And collectively it reflects the fact that mental health is unlike any other field we have encountered. It is a minefield.

In no other arena have we witnessed such disparate and strongly held views. Anti-psychiatry, pro-psychiatry, medical model versus social model, mental illness versus emotional crisis, medication versus compassionate listening . . .

Such debates have not been solved here, nor do we wish to solve them. We respect the opinions of everyone who spoke with us.

Amidst all these differing views, however, we have also discovered a common theme. It is, we believe, as crucial to recovery as medication or psychotherapy. We've titled our chapter after it. And it involves all of us.

First, we should point out that recovery does not mean cure. It instead denotes the ability to move on with our lives, past the stage where we view ourselves – and others us – as a "mental patient." It is about living again, in a world beyond diagnosis. About regaining our rightful role in society. And it is a message we first heard from a woman named Pat Capponi.

Pat is a psychiatric "survivor" – a term she uses to denote having "survived" the mental health system. She has emerged to become a potent voice, a powerful advocate, and a phenomenal writer. One of her books, *Upstairs in the Crazy House*, is a personal and searing account of her life after being diagnosed, impoverished, and discarded by "the system." It is a stark portrait of a world without hope, to which we abandon far too many. A place where human potential is forgotten, ignored.

I asked Pat, over lunch, what people with mental disorders need. The answer, just like the woman herself, was honest and to the point.

"A home, a job, a friend."

It was the first time we'd heard that phrase. And then we started talking to other people who'd been through the system. More importantly, we started listening.

A HOME

I met a lovely, older woman named Marilyn at a drop-in health clinic in downtown Toronto in November of 1997. It wasn't much of a clinic, really, but a kind doctor showed up every Tuesday afternoon to see whoever needed seeing. Some of the people came for reasons of physical health, some for psychiatric medication, some for both. All of them were poor, many were homeless.

Marilyn arrived for an injection of an antipsychotic drug she said helped keep some people called the Cabirs away. I asked her who the Cabirs were – and she showed me a bruised shoulder, said she'd been pushed down the stairs by one of the five Cabir brothers who lived with her. I was horrified that someone could abuse a sixty-four-year-old woman in such a way.

I asked Marilyn if she'd mind if I dropped by to visit. She seemed delighted that someone would actually take an interest in her.

Not long after that, I knocked on the door of a rooming house. It was home to many ex-psychiatric patients and was falling apart. Marilyn showed me into her room, a dimly lit hole with an old fridge and a silent, flickering black-and-white television. We sat down on chairs at the small table, the only furniture save for her bed. There was no sign of the Cabirs.

Before my eyes had fully adjusted to the dark, Marilyn smacked a tattered fly swatter down on the table. *Swaaaaap!* And again.

"Cockroaches," she said apologetically. *Swaaaaap!*

The table was crawling with them. Small ones, freshly hatched, were navigating between our cups, over my notebook, around the tape recorder. They were on the walls, in the carpet, everywhere. She'd told the landlord about them, she said, and about the nine mice she'd caught. Nothing had been done.

I asked about the Cabir brothers. She recalled one of many beatings she'd endured.

"He just went crazy and said, 'I hate you!'" she explained. "And he grabbed an ashtray and just – *pow!* – hit me over the head with it. Put his teeth in my face and was going for the knife . . ."

Marilyn started to weep at this vivid memory. Her recollection was so filled with detail that the Cabirs' actual location in the rooming house came as a shock.

"They're all in the wall," she said matter-of-factly. "They just stand there and keep giving me slurs all the time. They say I am very ugly. They say, 'I can't stand the sight of her.' Strange, isn't it?"

Marilyn has spent long periods of her adult life in a psychiatric hospital. She's also the kind of person who, despite her disorder, can function perfectly well in the community. The kind of person who has every *right* to live in the community – even if the Cabirs come along.

But the "community" we offered this aging woman was a shameful disgrace. In Toronto, where housing stock is unbelievably tight, Marilyn paid $330 per month for a decrepit, roach-infested hovel. A place so lonely and isolating it would test the sanity of anyone – let alone someone with a predisposition to hearing voices.

We have since seen many other examples of community. We have seen supportive housing that works – and many places that do not. We've heard the frustration of grown men and women who are tired of being denied the freedom to open the fridge for a snack. We've listened to the anger at being forced to share a tiny bedroom with a stranger in far worse shape than you. We've seen the stultifying boredom of having little to do but chain-smoke in the TV room. And we've heard, repeatedly, anecdotes of how such places drive people "crazy." Or keep them that way.

"We know the literature," a community psychiatrist stressed. "Environment can make such a difference."

In the spring of 1998, the City of Toronto took a look inside the building where Marilyn lived. Inspectors deemed it unfit for human habitation. Marilyn was hooked up with a mental health worker who was able to find for her – small miracle, this – a clean, subsidized apartment at $300 monthly. The worker later told me the infestation had been so bad that most of Marilyn's clothing, even her wig, was crawling with bugs. The professional was at pains to point out the psychological impact of living in such conditions.

"Can you imagine yourself [in such a place]?" she asked. "If I didn't have a decent place to go home to, I would be very ill. I would be crazy. I see people get really sick because they have unstable housing. . . . And I've seen how people can become very stabilized with their illness when they have decent housing and we're able to offer them some support.

"On a very, very fundamental level," she emphasized, "housing can make all the difference."

Marilyn seems much happier in her new place. It is clean, she has her own kitchen and bathroom, and feels safe. She says the surroundings have made a tremendous improvement in her mental health.

"Oh, 100% better," she smiled.

Yes, the Cabirs still visit.

But they're a lot easier to live with.

A JOB

Not too many legal administrators can say they've been in a psychiatric hospital in southern Thailand. But Sharon can. Not so long ago she found herself confined to a ward on the other side of the world. A place where breakfast was a fiery fish stew.

Sharon's difficulties began early. She was the eldest of five children with a mother who suffered from wild mood swings. She recalls her childhood as a period of "extreme sadness," followed, in her twenties, by bouts of depression.

Still, she somehow managed. Sometimes her disorder would be in check and jobs would last. Sometimes it would flare up and then the job was gone. But she always got by. In fact, she earned enough to pay for a long trip to Asia in 1987.

It was a mixed bag, that trip. While in the Tibetan capital of Lhasa, she witnessed a crackdown by the People's Liberation Army. She watched in disbelief as a number of civilians, including a young child, were shot.

She left Tibet soon after, eventually heading to southern Thailand and a relaxing beach resort. While there, however, her mood began to escalate. Before she (or anyone else) knew what was happening, she was delusional.

"I was convinced I was dead," she says, "that I just hadn't passed to the other side and was earthbound." Twice, messages inside her head told her to jump in the ocean to free herself.

Fellow travellers, concerned, quietly arranged for her to be hospitalized. They also notified the Canadian embassy in Bangkok that a young woman required their help.

Sharon eventually made it back home, where a preliminary diagnosis of bipolar affective disorder was confirmed. For the next several years she tried to keep working, freelancing, scraping by. But in 1995 her doctor recommended that she take two years away from work: the first for total rest, the second to ease back in. And that was the moment the true hell began.

"The day I was told to stop work," she says, pausing a moment, ". . . that was the worst day of my life. I realized it meant going on social assistance, less money, social stigma and self-stigma."

As Sharon's income dropped, she found she couldn't afford to socialize with friends. Going out to theatres and restaurants became a fading memory. Some of those close to her stopped calling, and she detected resentment from others – people who, because it wasn't a physical ailment, couldn't understand why she was off work. She gradually became more isolated, fuelling her depression.

"I couldn't do much of anything. I'd stay in bed or watch TV all day – just to block out the day."

Sharon found herself in a desperate situation. She needed the disability benefits in order to have her expensive medication paid for. Yet the gap on her resume was growing, and the drop in income was affecting other aspects of her life. She was not improving.

"I didn't have enough money to pay all the bills and eat properly," she says. "I lost a lot of weight and was susceptible to anything – flus, etc. – going around. The only good thing was that the drugs were paid for."

So great was her loss of self-esteem that she found herself avoiding new people or situations, intensifying her isolation.

"I came to dread meeting new people because of the inevitable questions: 'What do you do?' or 'Why aren't you working?' You're so much defined by what you do."

And then, after more than three years in this limbo, someone at a local Mood Disorders Association who knew of Sharon's legal expertise asked her a simple question. Would she like some part-time work? Though fearful she might fail, Sharon accepted. And slowly, but surely, things began to fall back into place.

"It did wonders for my self-esteem – and the extra money has made such a difference. It means I can buy more and better food. It means I can go out and socialize."

It also meant structure for a life that had been in a holding pattern. A reason to get dressed in the morning. A place to go. Something real to do. A task she takes pride in. Sharon's been working part-time now for a year and a half. Long enough that she's ready for the next step. To move back into the regular workforce. To put more distance between herself and her diagnosis.

"I used to let it define me: 'Sharon, manic-depressive, damaged goods,'" she says. "I used to despair of ever working again at a fulfilling, lucrative job. Being able to take a holiday again. Being able to be at a social gathering and say what I do for a living – and not have to hide it."

Data has shown that people who find meaningful employment spend fewer days in hospital and require fewer services than others. They also report, consistently, a better quality of life.

"Work is a highly symbolic method of including people in our society," observes John Trainor, a widely published authority on the impact of community supports on people who use psychiatric services.

"If someone is working, they are felt to be part of something. Whether it's a high job or a low job, it has a very strong social value."

Sharon knows that depression, perhaps even mania, may still dog her from time to time. That doesn't trouble her so much. Because she's recovered.

A FRIEND

Mario's been through a lot. He was only thirteen when he came to this country, a little Italian kid with defective kidneys.

At a time when he should have been making friends and adapting to his new life, Mario spent much of his time in hospital and in pain.

By his late teens, depression started slamming him like a sledgehammer every fall. Then, in his early twenties, he found himself psychotic and hospitalized – the first of roughly a dozen mental health admissions in his life. His family members were so shocked that he was in a psychiatric ward, they didn't know what to do.

"When someone goes crazy," he says, "they think you're going to be crazy for the rest of your life. People look at you strangely, differently."

Already delusional and frightened, he wasn't helped much by his family's discomfort. Yet he did meet someone during that first hospital stay who made a difference. She was a fellow patient – also of Italian heritage. She shared cigarettes with him, spent time talking, helped him come to terms with where he was and why.

"She'd calm me down, be there for me," he recalls. "She was kind – she was a saint."

That woman was the first of many saints Mario would encounter. On another occasion, it was a social worker – a guy named Dave who seemed to care about Mario more as a friend than as a client. During their first meeting, Mario remembers being so depressed he was unsure if he wanted to continue living.

"The first time meeting him, I was a real mess," he says. "And I was in tears. I said, 'Dave, I need your help. If you can't help me, I don't know what I'm going to do next.' And he said, 'Mario, hang in there. Don't give up – I'm gonna support you.' A true friend. There have been many people like David in my life."

People who listened when Mario needed to talk. Folks like the friend who encouraged Mario, at thirty, to return to school and attend a literacy program. People who stood by him through years of dialysis, operations, and his eventual kidney transplant. Friends who encouraged him to pursue his passion for poetry, sculpting, painting.

"I was totally lost, emotionally, psychologically, physically," he explains. "True friends help you. I had many good friends along the way who really understood me."

For Mario, it wasn't one single friend but a combination of friends who listened at critical times in his life. Some of those friends were fellow consumer/survivors, some were friends who'd stuck it out, some were even mental health professionals.

Six years ago, when he found a good psychotherapist, he truly found relief. This professional was less concerned with diagnosis than with "feelings and emotions" – and Mario discovered he had an abundance of both bottled up.

"My sessions were three or four hours. . . . I cried buckets," he says. "But that Pandora's box was finally opened." And as it opened, Mario began to make progress.

"I knew there was something at the end of this that was going to cure me. Not cure, *heal*."

He still finds it hard to hold back the tears when he describes the contribution friends have made to his life.

"Friends are people who see you as you are, make you feel that you have worth, that you have value," he observes. "That you're a human being like the rest of us."

Worth. Value. Validation. Their importance should not be underestimated.

William A. Anthony, the highly respected American authority on psychiatric rehabilitation, has written eloquently about the recovery process. One of his many papers appeared in the *Psychosocial Rehabilitation Journal* in 1993: "People who are recovering talk about the people who believed in them even when they did not believe in themselves, who encouraged their recovery but did not force it, who tried to listen and understand when nothing seemed to be making sense. Recovery is a deeply human experience, facilitated by the deeply human responses of others."

AND FINALLY . . .

We want you to finish this book, whether you're a consumer, survivor, family member, or professional, with hope. With the realization that recovery is not just possible, but probable – given the right supports.

Some of those supports will come from the medical world: drugs, therapy, doctors. But throughout this book we've tried to emphasize that recovery requires more than this. People need, and *deserve*, more in their lives. Meaningful friendships, fulfilling work or activity, a decent place to live: these are required elements in every recovery.

It's a fact forcefully stated more than a decade ago in "Mental Health For Canadians: Striking a Balance." The 1988 document was published by what was then Health and Welfare Canada. "The crucial point here," it reads, "is that mental disorder, even when serious and chronic, is never the only factor in determining mental health – it is but a single element within a much larger set of interconnected factors, all of which need to be addressed."

And what are some of those factors? The document listed several key problems that can keep people in a state of poor mental health. They include "rejection by friends, family or workmates . . . the stigma of mental illness . . . inability to find or keep suitable employment . . . lack of appropriate and affordable housing . . . "

The list goes on. But three of the top four reasons are the needs identified by Pat Capponi. Human needs. Determinants, in the truest sense, of mental health.

"Apart from their illness-related needs," states the report, *"people with mental disorders have the same range of mental health needs and aspirations as anyone else."*

We've added those italics for a reason. Because too often we become so preoccupied with the disorder that we forget that simple truth.

During the research and writing of this book, we've witnessed some pretty remarkable things. We've heard poetry so beautiful it made us weep, written and read by a woman with schizophrenia. We've seen a man with bipolar affective disorder finish law school, and thrive as a working lawyer. We've rolled with laughter at improvs put on by people with nearly every label in the DSM.

There's a beauty in seeing things like that. The misconceptions crumble. And you're left realizing that, when you forget about the disorder, these folks are just like everyone else. Just like you.

Recovery is a delicate, wonderful thing. Much like a flower, it needs nurturing. Care. Love.

We've been fortunate enough to witness it in our own household.

We hope and trust it will come to yours.

APPENDIX

If only we had room to note down every worthwhile organization. There are literally hundreds of them across the country, with varying philosophies, approaches, and memberships. But space permits us to name only a few, so consider the list below as simply a place to start.

You may need to make more than one phone call. For example, we've noted only the national and provincial offices of self-help groups, but most will have local chapters (ask for the one nearest you) and will be able to refer you to addiction, women's, and culturally sensitive agencies. Crisis and 24-hour help lines are listed on the front page of your local phone book.

Within categories, everything is listed alphabetically, so order does not indicate preference or importance.

NATIONAL ORGANIZATIONS

FEDERAL GOVERNMENT

Health Canada, A.L. 0913A, Ottawa, Ontario K1A 0K9. Phone: 613-957-2991 (general enquiries); 613-954-7802 (mental health services). Website: www.hc-sc.gc.ca.

Health Canada, Regional Offices (Communications offices can direct you to mental health services)

- Nova Scotia: Suite 702, Ralston Building, 1557 Hollis Street, Halifax B3J 3V4. Phone: 902-426-2038 (Communications).
- Quebec: Room 218, Complexe Guy-Favreau, East Tower, 200 René Lévesque Blvd. West, Montreal H2Z 1X4.
- Ontario: 25 St. Clair Avenue East, 4th Floor, Toronto M4T 1M2. Phone: 416-973-4389.
- Manitoba: 391 York Avenue, Suite 425, Winnipeg R3C 0P4. Phone: 204-983-2508 (Communications).
- Alberta: Suite 710, Canada Place, 9700 Jasper Avenue, Edmonton T5J 4C3. Phone: 780-495-2651.
- British Columbia: Suite 405, Winch Building, 757 West Hastings Street, Vancouver V6C 1A1. Phone: 604-666-2083.

PROFESSIONAL ASSOCIATIONS

Acupuncture Foundation of Canada Institute, 2131 Lawrence Ave. East, Suite 204, Scarborough, Ontario M1R 5G4. Phone: 416-752-3988. E-mail: info@afcinstitute.com. Website: www.afcinstitute.com.

Canadian Association of Occupational Therapists, CTTC Building, Suite 3400, 1125 Colonel By Drive, Ottawa, Ontario K1S 5R1. Phone: 613-523-2268; toll-free 1-800-434-2268. Website: www.caot.ca.

Canadian Association of Social Workers, #402 - 383 Parkdale Avenue, Ottawa, Ontario K1Y 4R4. Phone: 613-729-6668. E-mail: casw@casw-acts.ca.

Canadian Naturopathic Association, 1255 Sheppard Ave. East, North York,

Ontario M2K 1E2. Phone: 416-496-8633. E-mail: info@naturopathicassoc.ca. Website: www.naturopathicassoc.ca.

Canadian Nurses Association, 50 Driveway, Ottawa, Ontario K2P 1E2. Phone: 613-237-2133; toll-free 1-800-361-8404. Website: www.cna-nurses.ca.

Canadian Psychiatric Association, #260 - 441 MacLaren Street, Ottawa, Ontario K2P 2H3. Phone: 613-234-2815. E-mail: cpa@medical.org. Website: www.cpa-apc.org.

Canadian Psychological Association, 151 Slater Street, Ste. 205, Ottawa, Ontario K1P 5H3. Phone: 613-237-2144; toll-free 1-888-472-0657. Website: www.cpa.ca.

College of Family Physicians of Canada, 2630 Skymark Avenue, Mississauga, Ontario L4W 5A4. Phone: 905-629-0900. E-mail: info@cfpc.ca. Website: www.cfpc.ca.

Dietitians of Canada, 480 University Avenue, Suite 604, Toronto, Ontario M5G 1V2. Phone: 416-596-0857. E-mail: centralinfo@dietitians.ca. Website: www.dietitians.ca.

GP-Psychotherapy Association, 365 Bloor Street East, Ste. 1807, Toronto, Ontario M4W 3L4. Phone: 416-410-6644. E-mail: gppa@collinscan.com.

SELF-HELP GROUPS

Canadian Mental Health Association (CMHA), National Office, 2160 Yonge Street, 3rd Floor, Toronto, Ontario M4S 2Z3. Phone: 416-484-7750; toll-free 1-800-875-6213. E-mail: cmhanat@interlog.com. Website: www.cmha.ca.

The Mood Disorders Association of Canada, #4 - 1000 Notre Dame Avenue, Winnipeg, Manitoba R3E 0N3. Phone: 204-786-0987.

The National Eating Disorder Information Centre, CW 1-211, 200 Elizabeth Street, Toronto, Ontario M5G 2C4. Phone: 416-340-4156. E-mail: nedic@uhn.on.ca. Website: www.nedic.on.ca.

National Network for Mental Health, 55 King Street, Suite 303, St. Catharines, Ontario L2R 3H5. Phone: 905-682-2423; toll-free 1-888-406-4663. E-mail: member@nnmh.on.ca. Website: www.nnmh.on.ca.

Schizophrenia Society of Canada, 75 The Donway W., Suite 814, Don Mills, Ontario M3C 2E9. Phone: 416-445-8204; toll-free 1-888-772-4673. E-mail: info@schizophrenia.ca. Website: www.schizophrenia.ca.

SUICIDE RESOURCES (provide information only, not crisis services)

Canadian Association for Suicide Prevention, c/o The Support Network, #301, 11456 Jasper Avenue NW, Edmonton, Alberta T5K 0M1. Phone: 780-482-0198. E-mail: casp@suicideprevention.ca. Website: www.suicideprevention.ca.

Suicide Information & Education Centre, #201, 1615 10th Ave. SW, Calgary, Alberta T3C 0J7. Phone: 403-245-3900. E-mail: siec@siec.ca. Website: www.siec.ca.

SURVIVOR ORGANIZATIONS

Lunatics' Liberation Front, Box 3075, Vancouver, British Columbia V6B 3X6. E-mail: bat@walnet.org. Website: www.walnet.org/llf/index.html.

People Against Coercive Treatment (PACT). Phone: 416-760-2795. E-mail: pact@tao.ca. Website: www.tao.ca/~pact.

Psychiatric Survivor Action Association of Ontario. E-mail: saao@icomm.ca. Website: www.icomm.ca/psaao/.

Second Opinion Society (SOS), 708 Black Street, Whitehorse, Yukon Y1A 2N8. Phone: 867-667-2037. E-mail: sos@yukon.net.

PHONE SERVICES

DIRECT Depression Information Line (Taped information, 24 hours). Phone: toll-free 1-888-557-5051 (access code 8000). Website: www-fhs.mcmaster.ca/direct.

Kids Help Phone. Phone: toll-free 1-800-668-6868. Website: kidshelp.sympatico.ca.

Schizophrenia Society of Canada Help Line. Phone: toll-free 1-800-809-4673.

PROVINCIAL ORGANIZATIONS

BRITISH COLUMBIA

Government

Mental Health Advocate of B.C., #905 - 207 W. Hastings Street, Vancouver V6B 1H7. Phone: 604-775-4000; toll-free 1-877-222-0412. E-mail: mhinfo@mhadvocate.com. Website: www.mhadvocate.com.

Ministry of Health, 1515 Blanshard Street, Victoria V8W 3C8. Phone: 250-952-3456 (general inquiries). Website: www.hlth.gov.bc.ca. Public Health Infoline: toll-free 1-800-665-4347; Victoria 250-952-1742. Mental Health Information Line: toll-free 1-800-661-2121 (taped information); Vancouver 604-669-7600.

Professional Associations

B.C. Naturopathic Association. Phone: 604-736-6646

B.C. Psychological Association. Phone: 604-730-0522 (referral line); toll-free 1-800-730-0522. E-mail: bcpa@interchange.ubc.ca.

College of Physicians & Surgeons of B.C. Phone: 604-733-7758; toll-free 1-800-661-9701. E-mail: Questions@cpsbc.bc.ca. Website: www.cpsbc.bc.ca.

Self-Help Groups

British Columbia Schizophrenia Society, #201 - 6011 Westminster Highway, Richmond V7C 4V4. Phone: 604-270-7841. Website: www.bcss.org.

CMHA, B.C. Division, #1200 - 1111 Melville Street, Vancouver V6E 3V6. Phone: 604-688-3234. E-mail: office@cmha-bc.org. Website: www.cmha-bc.org.

Eating Disorder Resource Centre, 1081 Burrard Street, St. Paul's Hospital, 2nd Floor, Vancouver V6Z 1Y6. Phone: toll-free 1-800-665-1822; Vancouver 604-806-9000. E-mail: edrcbc@direct.ca.

Mood Disorders Association of British Columbia, #201 - 2730 Commercial Drive, Vancouver V5N 5P4. Phone: 604-873-0103. E-mail: mda@lynx.bc.ca. Website: www.lynx.bc.ca/~mda.

Self-Help Resource Association of B.C., #303 - 1212 West Broadway, Vancouver V6H 3V1. Phone: 604-733-6186.

ALBERTA
Government

Alberta Mental Health Board, P.O. Box 1360, 10025 Jasper Avenue, Edmonton T5J 2N3. Phone: toll-free 877-303-2642; Edmonton 780-422-2233. Website: www.amhb.ab.ca.

Mental Health Patient Advocate, 12th Floor, Ctr. W., 10035 108th Street, Edmonton T5J 3E1. Phone: 780-422-1812.

Ministry of Health. Phone: Edmonton 780-427-1432; Calgary 403-297-6411; toll-free for rest of Alberta 310-0000. E-mail: ahinform@health.gov.ab.ca. Website: www.health.gov.ab.ca.

Professional Associations

Alberta Association of Naturopathic Practitioners. Phone: 403-266-2446.

College of Physicians & Surgeons of Alberta. Phone: toll-free 1-800-561-3899; Edmonton 780-423-4764. Website: www.cpsa.ab.ca.

Psychologists' Association of Alberta. Phone: 780-424-0294 (referral line); toll-free 1-888-424-0297. E-mail: paa@psychologistsassociation.ab.ca. Website: www.psychologistsassociation.ab.ca.

Self-Help Groups

Alberta Mental Health Self-Help Network, 328 Capital Place, 9707 110th Street NW, Edmonton T5K 2L9. Phone: 780-482-6576. E-mail: network@abc.mha.ca.

CMHA, Alberta Division, 328 Capital Place, 9707 110th Street NW, Edmonton T5K 2L9. Phone: 780-482-6576. E-mail: division@cmha.ab.ca. Website: www.cmha.ab.ca.

Depression and Manic-Depression Association of Alberta, P.O. Box 64064, 11528 107th Avenue, Edmonton T5H 0X0. Phone: toll-free 1-888-757-7077. E-mail: goldlina@telusplanet.net. Website: www.incentre.net/dmdaa/home.html.

Schizophrenia Society of Alberta, 9942 108th Street, 5th Floor, Edmonton T5K 2J5. Phone: 780-427-0579; toll-free 1-800-661-4644. E-mail: ssaprovincial1@interbaum.com. Website: www.schizophrenia.ca/abprov.html.

Society for Assisted Cooperative Recovery from Eating Disorders, Room 405, 10830 Jasper Avenue, Edmonton T5J 2B3.

SASKATCHEWAN
Government

Saskatchewan Health, Community Care Branch, 3475 Albert Street, Regina S4S 6X6. Phone: 306-787-3297. Website: www.gov.sk.ca/health.

Professional Associations

College of Physicians & Surgeons of Saskatchewan. Phone: 306-244-7355. Website: cpss@quadrant.net.

Saskatchewan Psychological Association. Phone: 306-955-3588. E-mail: spa@sk.sympatico.ca.

Self-Help Groups

CMHA, Saskatchewan Division, 2702 12th Avenue, Regina S4T 1J2. Phone: 306-525-5601. E-mail: cmhask@cmhask.com. Website: www.cmhask.com.

Schizophrenia Society of Saskatchewan, 400 Broad Street, Regina S4R IX3. Mailing Address: P.O. Box 305, Regina S4P 3AI. Phone: 306-584-2620. E-mail: ssprov@sk.sympatico.ca. Website: www.t2.net/schsask.

MANITOBA
Government

Ministry of Health, 300 Carlton Street, Winnipeg R3B 3M9. Phone: 204-786-7101 (general info); 204-788-6659 (Mental Health Program); 204-788-6782 (Mental Health Review Board); toll-free 1-877-218-0102. Website: www.gov.mb.ca/health.

Professional Associations

College of Physicians & Surgeons of Manitoba. Phone: 204-774-4344. Website: www.umanitoba.ca/colleges/cps/.

Manitoba Psychological Society. Phone: 204-488-7398. Website: www.mps.mb.ca.

Self-Help Groups

Anxiety Disorders Association of Manitoba, 825 Sherbrook Street, Winnipeg R3A IM5. Phone: toll-free 1-800-805-8885; Winnipeg 204-925-0600.

CMHA, Manitoba Division, #2 - 836 Ellice Avenue, Winnipeg R3G 0C2. Phone: 204-775-8888. E-mail: cmhaman@mb.imag.net. Website: www.cmhamanitoba.mb.ca.

Manitoba Schizophrenia Society, #3 - 1000 Notre Dame Avenue, Winnipeg R3E 0N3. Phone: 204-786-1616; toll-free 1-800-263-5545. E-mail: info@mss.mb.ca. Website: www.mss.mb.ca.

Manitoba Self-Help Clearing House, 825 Sherbrook Street, Winnipeg R3A IM5. Phone: 204-772-6979.

Mood Disorders Association of Manitoba, #4 - 1000 Notre Dame Avenue, Winnipeg R3E 0N3. Phone: 204-786-0987; toll-free 1-800-263-1460. E-mail: sdmdm@depression.mb.ca. Website: www.depression.mb.ca.

ONTARIO
Government

Centre for Addiction and Mental Health, 250 College Street, Toronto M5T IR8. Phone: 416-535-8501. Website: www.camh.net.

Ministry of Health, 5700 Yonge Street, 5th Floor, Toronto M2M 4K5. Phone: 416-327-7239 (Mental Health Unit); 416-327-4327 (Health INFOline); toll-free 1-800-268-1154. Website: www.gov.on.ca/health/english/program/mental.

Psychiatric Patient Advocate Office, 2195 Yonge Street, 6th Floor, Toronto M4S 2B2. Phone: 416-327-7000; toll-free 1-800-578-2343. E-mail:ppao@gov.on.ca. Website: www.ppao.gov.on.ca.

Professional Associations

College of Physicians and Surgeons of Ontario. Phone: 416-967-2626 (referrals); toll-free 1-800-268-7096. Website: www.cpso.on.ca.

Ontario Naturopathic Association. Phone: 416-233-2001.

Ontario Psychiatric Association. Phone: 905-827-4659.

Ontario Psychological Association. Phone: 416-961-0069 (referrals); toll-free 1-800-268-0069. E-mail: opa@psych.on.ca. Website: www.psych.on.ca.

Self-Help Groups

Anxiety Disorders Association of Ontario, 797 Somerset Street West, Suite 14, Ottawa K1R 6R3. Phone: 613-729-6761; toll-free 1-877-308-3843. E-mail: contactus@anxietyontario.com. Website: www.anxietyontario.com.

CMHA, **Ontario Division,** 180 Dundas St. West, Ste. 2301, Toronto M5G 1Z8. Phone: 416-977-5580; toll-free 1-800-875-6213. E-mail: division@ontario.cmha.ca. Website: www.ontario.cmha.ca.

Consumer/Survivor Development Initiative, 2160 Yonge Street, 3rd Floor, Toronto M4S 2Z3. Phone: 416-484-8785. E-mail: csdi@csdinit.on.ca. Website: www.csdinit.on.ca.

Mood Disorders Association of Ontario and Toronto, 40 Orchard View Blvd., Ste. 222, Toronto M4R 1B9. Phone: 416-486-8046; toll-free 1-888-486-8236. E-mail: mdamt@sympatico.ca. Website: www3. sympatico.ca/mdamt.

Northern Initiative for Social Action (NISA), 680 Kirkwood Drive, Building 2, Sudbury P3E 1X3. Phone: 705-675-9193, ext. 8206. E-mail: info@nisa.on.ca. Website: www.nisa.on.ca.

Ontario Council of Alternative Businesses, 761 Queen Street West, Rm. 307, Toronto M6J 1G1. Phone: 416-504-1693. E-mail: ocab@icomm.ca. Website: www.icomm.ca/ocab.

Ontario Self Help Network, 40 Orchard View Blvd., Ste. 219, Toronto M4R 1B9. Phone: 416-487-4355; toll-free 1-888-283-8806. E-mail: online@selfhelp.on.ca. Website: www.selfhelp.on.ca.

Schizophrenia Society of Ontario, 885 Don Mills Road, Ste. 322, Don Mills M3C 1V9. Phone: 416-449-6830; toll-free 1-800-449-6367. E-mail: sso@web.net. Website: www.schizophrenia.on.ca.

Phone Lines

CMHA **Information and Referral line** (Toronto). Phone: 416-789-7957.

Gerstein Centre (crisis service). Phone: 416-929-5200. E-mail: gerstein.ctr@sympatico.ca. Website: worldchat.com/public/tab/gerstein/gerstein.htm.

Info-Ability (information on services/resources). Phone: toll-free 1-800-665-9092.

QUEBEC

Government

Ministère de la Santé et des Services Sociaux, 1075, chemin Sainte Foy, 15e étage, Quebec G1S 2M1. Phone: 418-643-3380 (general info); toll-free 1-800-707-3380. Website: www.msss.gouv.gc.ca.

Professional Associations

Association des Médecins Psychiatres du Québec. Phone: 514-350-5128.

Collège des Médecins du Québec. Phone: 514-933-4441; toll-free 1-888-633-3246. E-mail: info@cmq.org. Website: www.cmq.org.

Ordre des Psychologues du Québec (OPQ). Phone: 514-738-1223;

toll-free 1-800-561-1223. E-mail: sercomm@ordrepsy.qc.ca. Website: www.ordrepsy.qc.ca.

Regroupement des ressources alternatives en santé mentale du Québec Inc. (RRASMQ). Phone: 514-523-7919.

Self-Help Groups

AMI-**Québec Alliance for the Mentally Ill,** 5253 Decarie Blvd., Ste. 150, Montreal H3W 3C3. Phone: 514-486-1448. E-mail: amique@dsuper.net. Website: www.dsuper.net/~amique.

Association canadienne pour la santé mentale (CMHA), 550, rue Sherbrooke Ouest, Ste. 2075, Montreal H3A 1B9. Phone: 514-849-3291. Website: www.cam.org/acsm. E-mail: acsm@cam.org.

L'Association des Dépressifs et Maniaco-Dépressifs, 801, rue Sherbrook Est, Bur. 500, Montreal H2L 1K7. Phone: 514-529-7552; 514-529-5619 (help line). E-mail: admd@cam.org.

L' Association des groupes d'interventions en défense de droits en santé mentale du Québec (AGIDO-SMQ), 4837, rue Boyer, Ste. 210, Montreal H2J 3E6. Phone: 514-523-3443. E-mail: agidd@cam.org.

L'Association Québécoise de la Schizophrénie, 7401, rue Hochelago, Montreal H1N 3M5. Phone: 514-251-4000, ext. 3400. Website: www.schizophrenia.ca/pqprov.html.

Association Québécoise de suicidologie inc., 800, boul. St-Joseph Est, Montreal H2J 1K4. Phone: 514-528-5858. E-mail: aqs@cam.org.

Fédération des familles et amis de la personne atteinte de maladie mentale (FFAPAMM), 1990, rue Jean-Talon Nord, bur. 203, Sainte-Foy G1N 4K8. Phone: 418-687-0474; toll-free 1-800-323-0474. E-mail: FFAPMM@qc.aina.com.

NEW BRUNSWICK

Government

Family and Community Services, P.O. Box 5001, 300 St. Mary Street, Fredericton E3B 5G4. Phone: 506-453-3953; 506-453-2132 (Mental Health Services Division); toll-free 1-800-442-9799 (after-hours emergency service). Website: www.gov.nb.ca/hcs-ssc.

New Brunswick Patient Advocate Services, 115 Connaught Avenue, Moncton E1C 3P4. Phone: 506-856-2924.

Professional Associations

College of Physicians and Surgeons of New Brunswick. Phone: 506-849-5050; toll-free 1-800-667-4641. E-mail: info@cpsnb.org. Website: www.cpsnb.org.

College of Psychologists of New Brunswick. Phone: 506-459-1994. E-mail: cpnb@nbnet.nb.ca.

Self-Help Groups

CHIMO. Phone: 506-450-4357 (helpline); toll-free 1-800-667-5005 (helpline).

CMHA, **New Brunswick Division,** 65 Brunswick Street, Suite 292, Fredericton E3B 1G5. Phone: 506-455-5231. E-mail:

cmhanb@nbnet.nb.ca. Website: www.unb.ca/web/netlearn/english/ c/cmha-nb/index.shtml.

New Brunswick Mental Health Consumer Network, 116 Martin Street, Edmundston E3V 2M9. Phone: 506-735-4442.

Schizophrenia Society of New Brunswick, P.O. Box 562, Miramichi E1V 3T7. Phone: 506-622-1595. Website: www.schizophrenia.ca/ nbprov.html.

NOVA SCOTIA
Government

Department of Health, P.O. Box 488, Joseph Howe Bldg., 1690 Hollis, Halifax B3J 2R8. Phone: 902-424-5818 (general info); toll-free 1-800-387-6665. Website: www.gov.ns.ca/health.

Health Services by Region: Central Region, 902-460-6840; Northern Region, 902-897-6265; Eastern Region, 902-794-6010; Western Region, 902-638-3452.

Professional Associations

Association of Psychologists of Nova Scotia. Phone: 902-422-9183. E-mail: apns@ns.sympatico.ca. Website: www3.ns.sympatico.ca/apns.

College of Physicians and Surgeons of Nova Scotia. Phone: 902-422-5823; toll-free 1-877-282-7767. Website: www.cpsns.ns.ca.

Self-Help Groups

CMHA, Nova Scotia Division, 63 King Street, Dartmouth B2Y 2R7. Phone: 902-466-6600. E-mail: cmhans@netcom.ca. Website: www.cmhans.com.

Depressive and Manic Depressive Society of Nova Scotia, c/o 73 Howe Street, Sydney B1P 4T9.

Schizophrenia Society of Nova Scotia, P.O. Box 1004, Room 409, Simpson Hall, Nova Scotia Hospital, Dartmouth B2Y 3Z9. Phone: 902-465-2601; toll-free 1-800-465-2601. E-mail: ssns@ns.sympatico.ca.

Self-Help Connection, 63 King Street, Dartmouth B2Y 2R7. Phone: 902-466-2011. E-mail: self-help@chebucto.ns.ca. Website: www.chebucto.ns.ca/community/support/SHC.

PRINCE EDWARD ISLAND
Government

Department of Health and Social Services, 16 Garfield Street, P.O. Box 2000, Charlottetown C1A 7N8. Phone: 902-368-6130; 902-368-6718 (Mental Health Consultant). Website: www.gov.pe.ca/infopei/Health.

Health Information Resource Centre, 1 Rochford Street (Charlottetown Area Health Centre), P.O. Box 2000, Charlottetown C1A 7N8. Phone: 902-368-6526; toll-free 1-800-241-6971.

Professional Associations

PEI College of Physicians and Surgeons. Phone: 902-566-3861.

PEI Psychiatric Association. Phone: 902-368-4430.

PEI Psychologists Registration Board. Phone: 902-566-0310.
Psychological Association of PEI. Phone: 902-368-4430.
Self-Help Groups
   CMHA, Prince Edward Island Division, 178 Fitzroy St., P.O. Box 785,
      Charlottetown C1A 7L9. Phone: 902-566-3034. E-mail:
      cmhapei@bigfoot.com. Website: www3.pei.sympatico.ca/cmha.
   Schizophrenia Society of PEI, P.O. Box 785, 178 Fitzroy St.,
      Charlottetown C1A 7L9. Phone: 902-566-5573. E-mail:
      info@schizophreniaPEI.pe.ca.Website: www.schizophreniapei.pe.ca.
   Self-Help Clearinghouse, 178 Fitzroy Street, P.O. Box 785,
      Charlottetown, C1A 7N8. Phone: 902-628-1648; toll-free
      1-800-682-1648.

NEWFOUNDLAND & LABRADOR
Government
   Mental Health Crisis Centre (24-hour service), 47 St. Clare Avenue, St.
      John's A1C 2J9. Phone: 709-737-4668; toll-free 1-888-737-4668.
   Ministry of Health and Community Services, 20 Cordage Place, P.O.
      Box 13122, St. John's A1B 4A4. Phone: 709-738-4922 (Mental
      Health line). Website: public.gov.nf.ca/health.
Professional Associations
   Association of Newfoundland Psychologists. Phone: 709-739-5405.
      E-mail: hcc.nicjo@hccsj.nf.ca.
   Newfoundland Board of Examiners in Psychology. Phone: 709-
      579-6313.
   Newfoundland Medical Board. Phone: 709-726-8546.
Self-Help Groups
   Channal, P.O. Box 5788, 354 Water Street, St. John's A1C 5X3. Phone:
      709-753-5111.
   CMHA, Newfoundland Division, 354 Water St., 3rd Floor, St. John's
      A1C 5X3. Phone: 709-753-8550. E-mail: cmha@nfld.com. Website:
      www.nflab.cmha.ca/.
   Schizophrenia Society of Newfoundland and Labrador, 6 Woodford
      Place, Mount Pearl A1N 2S2. Phone: 709-745-7765. Website:
      www.schizophrenia.ca/nfldprov.html.

YUKON
Government
   Health and Social Services, Box 2703, Whitehorse Y1A 2C6. Phone:
      867-667-8346 (Mental Health Services); toll-free 1-800-661-0408.
      Website: www.hss.gov.yk.ca.
Professional Groups
   Yukon Medical Council. Phone: 867-667-5111.
Self-Help Groups
   CMHA, Yukon Division, 6 Bates Crescent, Whitehorse Y1A 4T8. Phone:
      867-668-8812

NORTHWEST TERRITORIES
Government
> **Health and Social Services,** Box 1320, Yellowknife X1A 2L9. Phone: 867-873-7991 (Community Programs and Services); 867-873-7926 (Mental Health Consultant). E-mail: health@gov.nt.ca. Website: www.hlthss.gov.nt.ca.

Professional Associations
> **Association of Psychologists of the Northwest Territories.** Phone: 867-873-8170.
> **The Northwest Territories Medical Association.** Phone: 867-920-4575.

Self-Help Groups
> CMHA, **Northwest Territories Division,** P.O. Box 2580, Suite 204, 5102 50th Avenue., Yellowknife X1A 2P9. Phone: 867-873-3190. E-mail: cmha@yk.com. CMHA Help Line: 867-920-2121; toll-free 1-800-661-0844.

NUNAVUT
Government
> **Department of Health and Social Services,** Box 800, Iqaluit, Nunavut X0A 0H0. Phone: 867-975-5700.
> Health and Social Services Boards: Baffin Region (Iqaluit), 867-979-7601; Keewatin Region (Rankin Inlet), 867-645-2171; Kitikmeot Region (Cambridge Bay), 867-983-7328.

Professional Associations
> **Association of Psychologists of the Northwest Territories.** Phone: 867-873-8170.
> **Northwest Territories Medical Association.** Phone: 867-920-4575.

GLOSSARY

Throughout this book, we've tried to explain clinical terms or potentially unfamiliar words as they arise. Here are a few we didn't get to in the text.

Anxiolytics are medications used to reduce anxiety. Most often the term "anxiolytics" refers to drugs in the benzodiazapine class. (See Chapter 8.)

Ayurvedic medicine is a holistic approach to health care that originated in India. Practitioners believe there are three types of energy, which exist in varying levels in each person's body, mind, and spirit. The key to good health is to keep these energies in balance. Practitioners look at the pulse, skin, tongue, and eyes to assess imbalances; treatment may include use of herbs, exercise, and changes in diet and lifestyle.

A **consumer** is a person who uses mental health services. Though it's a less-than-ideal term which some people reject, it is commonly used in the mental health field throughout North America. (In Britain, the term "user" is common.)

Controlled study refers to a scientific experiment involving at least two groups of people (or animals, or even bacteria). One group receives some kind of treatment or intervention, while the other (the control group) does not. The results between the two are then compared, providing researchers with evidence of what a particular treatment does or doesn't do. In a placebo-controlled trial, a pill or procedure of no clinical value is given to the control group.

Crazy-making is any external event or situation that people with mental health issues find particularly troublesome. Being stigmatized, living in poverty, sitting alone in a room all day, or dealing with bureaucracies – these are all examples of the many things that can make a person feel "crazy."

A **depot** is a long-lasting injection of antipsychotic medication. The drug is released slowly in your system for a period of two weeks to a month. Some people, particularly those who have difficulty remembering to take medication on a daily basis, prefer this method.

Dietitians have university degrees in food and nutrition and are trained to help people improve their health by altering their diets. They can assess what you eat, identify problems, and develop diet plans, either to meet specific medical conditions or for overall health. Registered dietitians work in hospitals and other health care facilities, although some work in private practice.

Endogenous means "originating from within the body." An endogenous depression, for example, might be triggered by a thyroid problem, with life events playing no significant role.

Hypnotic refers to a group of drugs used to induce sleep. Most hypnotics achieve this by temporarily depressing the central nervous system.

Lack of insight is a phrase usually used to indicate that a person with a disorder does not fully appreciate the severity of that disorder – or even its existence. Someone who repeatedly has severe psychotic episodes, yet fails to understand or accept the need for medication, would be said to lack insight. It should be noted that this can be a controversial term, especially for psychiatric "survivors" (see below) who think it's falsely used against anyone who challenges a doctor's diagnosis.

Naturopathic medicine uses herbs, vitamins, homeopathic remedies, and other natural products – as well as dietary and lifestyle changes – to enhance natural healing. Naturopathic doctors are highly trained and tailor treatment plans to each individual after a comprehensive diagnostic interview. Their services may be covered by private health plans.

Neuroleptics are more commonly known as antipsychotics. These are medications used to keep psychosis at bay and are most often used with schizophrenia. *Barron's Dictionary of Medical Terms* describes such drugs as causing neurolepsis, an "altered state of consciousness marked by indifference to the surroundings; quiescence."

Occupational therapists help clients develop practical living skills like budgeting, shopping, and scheduling, and link them up with community and recreational services. Their goal is to help people live more independent, fulfilling lives. Occupational therapists have university degrees and work in hospitals, community health, and home-care programs; your family doctor can provide a referral. Their services are covered by provincial health plans.

A **placebo** is an inert, clinically insignificant pill or procedure used in controlled studies (see above). Subjects in such a study do not know whether they're receiving, say, a genuine antidepressant or merely a capsule that looks like one. Interestingly, studies have consistently found that, on average, one-third of the people receiving the fake treatment show some improvement; this is called "the placebo effect." For a treatment or procedure to be considered effective, it must do better than the placebo did in that study.

Prophylactic treatments are taken not to quell symptoms but to prevent them from returning. Someone with a history of chronic depressive episodes, for example, might take antidepressants, even when their mood is fine, in the hope of preventing a future episode.

Psychosis is a state of mind where one has lost touch with reality. Psychosis can involve delusions, hallucinations, paranoia, and other abnormal thought processes. These thoughts and altered perceptions are very real to the psychotic person. Psychosis is usually associated with major mental disorders, but can also be induced through sleep deprivation.

Psychotropic is the word used to describe any mind- or mood-altering drug. In the mental health world, it covers virtually the entire range of psychotherapeutic medications. It can also be used to describe drugs such as crack or LSD.

Remission is something we all look forward to. It's the partial or complete disappearance of symptoms in either a mental or physical disorder. Even in cases where the symptoms vanish, the underlying disorder is still considered to be present. Remission can occur either as a response to treatment or spontaneously.

Suicidal ideation involves dwelling, constantly or frequently, on thoughts of ending one's life. Even if the person tries to banish such thoughts, they can still pop spontaneously into their mind. This ideation often involves the graphic visualizing of specific methods of suicide, and is common in cases of extreme depression.

Survivor is as much a political term as anything else. People who have had unpleasant experiences with psychiatry often feel they have "survived" the mental health system. Some survivors reject the medical model upon which psychiatry is based and do not believe in the existence of mental disorder.

Traditional Chinese medicine is a centuries-old system that uses acupuncture, herbs, and massage to achieve and maintain health. Mind and body are not separated as they are in Western medicine; practitioners treat the whole person by balancing their energy, or *Qi*. Traditional medicine is still widely used in China; practitioners are university educated and hold doctoral degrees.

Trauma refers to psychological and emotional wounds caused by some form of assault or abuse. These include physical or sexual abuse, and life-threatening events such as war, torture, or violent crime. Trauma research is a relatively new field; clinicians and researchers are still exploring the relationship between trauma and mental disorder.

USEFUL BOOKS

Throughout this book, we've tried to give you a sense of the range of opinions, experiences, and perspectives relating to mental health. The following list reflects that diversity; you won't necessarily agree with everything you read in these books, but you'll learn something from each of them. We've read all of these books, and have referred to many of them in earlier chapters. Yet the list is, of necessity, incomplete; we encourage you to dig around at libraries and bookstores. Also look for brochures published by self-help groups like the CMHA – they generally provide useful, practical information for both consumers and family members.

Books marked with an asterisk (*) are Canadian.

PERSONAL STORIES

A Brilliant Madness: Living with Manic-Depressive Illness, by Patty Duke and Gloria Hochman. New York: Bantam Books, 1992.

Darkness Visible: A Memoir of Madness, by William Styron. New York: Vintage Books, 1990.

Holiday of Darkness: A Psychologist's Personal Journey Out of His Depression, by Norman S. Endler. Toronto: Wall & Thompson, 1990.

In the Jaws of the Black Dogs: A Memoir of Depression, by John Bentley Mays. Toronto: Penguin Books, 1995.

An Unquiet Mind: A Memoir of Moods and Madness, by Kay Redfield Jamison. New York: Alfred A. Knopf, 1996.

Upstairs in the Crazy House: The Life of a Psychiatric Survivor, by Pat Capponi. Toronto: Viking, 1992.

REFERENCE WORKS

Alternative Medicine: What Works, by Adriane Fugh-Berman. Baltimore: Williams & Wilkins, 1997.

The Broken Brain: The Biological Revolution in Psychiatry, by Nancy Andreasen. New York: Harper & Row, 1984.

Caring for the Mind: The Comprehensive Guide to Mental Health, by Dianne Hales and Robert Hales. New York: Bantam Books, 1996.

A History of Psychiatry, by Dr. Edward Shorter. New York: John Wiley & Sons, 1997.

Living and Working with Schizophrenia, by J.J. Jeffries, E. Plummer, M. Seeman, J.F. Thornton. Toronto: University of Toronto Press, 1990.

Mental Illness: Opposing Viewpoints, edited by William Barbour. San Diego: Greenhaven Press, 1995.

Mindsets, Mental Health: The Ultimate Productivity Weapon, by Edgardo Pérez and Bill Wilkerson. Guelph: The Homewood Centre, 1998.

Molecules of Emotion: The Science Behind Mind-Body Medicine, by Candace B. Pert. New York: Simon & Schuster, 1997.

Overcoming Depression, revised edition, by Demitri Papolos and Janice Papolos. New York: HarperPerennial, 1997.

Partners in Healing: Perspectives on the Experience of Psychiatry, by Alan Eppel, Judity MacKay, Sheryl Pedersen and Tunde Szathmary. Hamilton: McMaster University Press, 1999.

The Seduction of Madness, by Edward M. Podvoll. New York: HarperCollins, 1990.

A Social History of Madness: Stories of the Insane, by Roy Porter. London: Weidenfeld and Nicholson, 1987.

Stress & Natural Healing, by Christopher Hobbs. Loveland: Interweave Press, 1997.

The Talking Cure, by Susan C. Vaughan. New York: Henry Holt, 1997.

Understanding & Treating Mental Illness, by John M. Cleghorn. Toronto: Hogrefe & Huber, 1991.

Women and Madness, by Phyllis Chesler. New York: Four Walls Eight Windows, 1997.

You Are Not Alone: A Handbook. Toronto: Mood Disorders Association of Metropolitan Toronto, 2000.

ANTI-PSYCHIATRY BOOKS

Call Me Crazy: Stories From the Mad Movement, by Irit Shimrat. Vancouver: Press Gang, 1997.

The Myth of Mental Illness, by Thomas S. Szasz. New York: Harper & Row, 1974.

Shrink Resistant: The Struggle Against Psychiatry in Canada, edited by Bonnie Burstow and Don Weitz. Vancouver: New Star Books, 1988.

Toxic Psychiatry, by Peter R. Breggin. New York: St. Martin's Press, 1991.

FOR FAMILIES

Contagious Emotions: Staying Well When Your Loved One Is Depressed, by Ronald M. Podell. New York: Pocket Books, 1992

Grieving Mental Illness: A Guide for Patients and Their Caregivers, by Virginia Lafond. Toronto: University of Toronto Press, 1994.

Helping Someone with Mental Illness: A Compassionate Guide for Family, Friends and Caregivers, by Rosalynn Carter. New York: Times Books, 1998.

Imagining Robert: My Brother, Madness, and Survival, by Jay Neugeboren. New York: Henry Holt, 1997.

My Brother Peter, by Nomi Berger. Montreal: Robert Davies, 1998.

Schizophrenia: A Handbook for Families. Ottawa: Department of National Health & Welfare in co-operation with the Schizophrenia Society of Canada, 1991.

When Someone You Love Has a Mental Illness: A Handbook for Family, Friends, and Caregivers, by Rebecca Woolis. New York: Putnam, 1992.

When Someone You Love Is Depressed, by Laura Epstein Rosen and Xavier Francisco Amador. New York: The Free Press, 1996.

MEDICAL TEXTS

The Canadian Medical Association Guide to Prescription and Over-the-Counter Drugs, edited by Mark S. Berner and Gerald N. Rotenberg. Montreal: The Reader's Digest Association (Canada), 1990.

Compendium of Pharmaceuticals and Specialties (CPS): The Canadian Reference for Health Professionals, 31st edition. Ottawa: Canadian Pharmaceutical Association, 1996.

Diagnostic Criteria From DSM-IV. Washington: American Psychiatric Association, 1998.

DSM-IV, The Diagnostic and Statistical Manual of Mental Disorders, 4th edition, American Psychiatric Association, 1994.

DSM-IV Made Easy: The Clinician's Guide to Diagnosis, by James Morrison. New York: The Guildford Press, 1995.

Psychiatric Diagnosis, 5th edition, by Donald W. Goodwin and Samuel B. Guze. New York: Oxford University Press, 1996.

USEFUL WEBSITES

There's a wonderful world of websites out there – if you have access to a computer, you can instantly connect with consumers, survivors, doctors, and mental health organizations anywhere on the planet. Within this world, you'll find online chat rooms, magazines, book reviews, and journal abstracts. In fact, there's so much out there the search can be overwhelming. Here are just a few places to start. These sites all provide useful information and should offer links to other websites.

CANADIAN SITES

Canadian Health Network – www.canadian-health-network.ca (Health Canada site covering all aspects of health, including mental health).